1993

CREATING NEW
HOSPITAL-PHYSICIAN
COLLABORATION

AMERICAN COLLEGE OF HEALTHCARE EXECUTIVES MANAGEMENT SERIES

Anthony R. Kovner, Series Editor

Todd S. Wirth and Seth Allcorn

CREATING NEW HOSPITAL-PHYSICIAN COLLABORATION

MANAGEMENT SERIES
American College of Healthcare Executives

97 96 95 94 93   5 4 3 2 1

Library of Congress Cataloging-in-Publication Data

Wirth, Todd S.
  Creating new hospital-physician collaboration / Todd S. Wirth, Seth Allcorn.
      p.   cm. — (Management series / American College of Healthcare Executives)
  Includes bibliographical references and index.
  ISBN 0-910701-96-2 (hardbound : alk. paper)
  1. Hospital-physician joint ventures.   2. Hospital-physician relations—Economic aspects.   3. Hospital mergers.   I. Allcorn, Seth.   II. Title.   III. Series: Management series (Ann Arbor, Mich.)
  [DNLM: 1. Hospital-Physician Joint Ventures—organization & administration.   2. Health Facility Merger—organization & administration.   WX 157 W799c 1993]
  RA410.58.W57   1993   362.1'1'068—dc20
  DNLM/DLC for Library of Congress   93-12245 CIP

The paper used in this publication meets the minimum requirements of American National Standard for Information Sciences—Permanence of Paper for Printed Library Materials, ANSI Z39.48-1984. ∞™

Health Administration Press
A division of the Foundation of the
  American College of Healthcare Executives
1021 East Huron Street
Ann Arbor, Michigan 48104-9990
(313) 764-1380

CONTENTS

147,122

FOREWORD

As the winds of health care reform blow ever stronger in the United States, scholars, policymakers, and health care providers are examining the health care delivery system in greater detail and with more attention to new concepts than ever before. One of the encouraging signs that reform can and will be accomplished is the growing number of publications by health care practitioners on new concepts and new ideas about how the delivery system can be changed and adapted to new policy requirements. This book represents just such a contribution from two experienced health care practitioners.

The focus of this work is a discussion of different methods hospitals and physicians can use and are using to integrate their efforts and organizations. An excellent foundation for the later chapters is developed for the reader with discussions on the economics of medical practice, the health care market, and the new controls on health care delivery emerging today. The development of medical groups and their growing importance to hospitals are also important parts of the foundation.

Based in part on their own experience, the authors describe why hospitals and physicians can work more effectively by working together than by pursuing their interests separately. They go on to suggest some practical concerns regarding the development of new organizational ventures between hospitals and physicians, which both groups must address if these ventures are to succeed.

The sections describing how medical groups govern themselves and approaches to assessing medical group operations will be useful to any reader. The description of the leadership politics of medical groups is informative for any reader, particularly those who are not directly involved in medical group management. The physician leadership style classification and the section on the psychological view of physician executives provide hospital executives and others with a way of understanding physician executive behavior.

Specific approaches to hospital-physician affiliation are described, as are the issues of governance, management, and financial arrangements. Hospital–medical group practice management service agreements are discussed with words of advice and caution. The authors show how agreements such as purchasing agreements, laboratory and radiology services, and space leasing can be steps hospitals and physicians use to begin their affiliation. The chapter on shared ownership of medical practices by hospitals is likely to be of great interest, given the current environment for health care. As the authors state, "Hospital involvement in the ownership of medical groups is one of the fastest growing trends in the hospital industry." Indeed, this is true, and the authors' writings on the topic are worth reading by any hospital or physician executive interested in this relationship. Topics such as organization structure, governance, patterns for problem solving, and financial issues are discussed.

The book will certainly be of greatest benefit to physicians, medical groups, and hospital executives interested in examining affiliations between physicians and hospitals. They will find the writings to be very practical and based on a good deal of experience. Useful examples of contracts, agreements, and other written materials are included. The authors offer a balanced description of the many issues related to hospitals and physicians as they come together in different forms of affiliation. The book is comprehensive, offering useful advise on how medical groups and hospitals can deal with these two groups who historically have remained independent of each other in the complex health care delivery system in the United States. The book will also provide many other readers with a greater understanding of the issues involved in integrating two of the provider elements in the U.S. health care delivery system.

Donald C. Wegmiller
Vice Chairman and President
HealthSpan Corporation

PREFACE

The growth of interest in integrating hospitals with medical groups is a new phenomenon on the American health care scene. Rising from virtual obscurity in the 1980s, hospital-physician networks are now expected to play an important role in the delivery of health care in the United States during the 1990s and beyond.

The networks promise greater size and complexity, which can threaten to outpace the development of effective means for their administration. The management of these networks will require the development of new methods. This book contributes to the development of the management knowledge and methods that will be needed to operate hospital-physician networks that must deal with the conflicting interests of (1) physicians who might have little knowledge of or often respect for hospital administrators, (2) rising costs that society hopes will be curbed, (3) increasing competition for patients, and (4) increasing reimbursement and regulatory complexity.

This book takes into consideration these influences. Every effort has been made to provide useful information to hospital administrators who wish to network with medical groups. The authors of this book hope that it will contribute to this new and demanding area of endeavor that will require the very best from health care services managers.

ACKNOWLEDGMENTS

We wish to acknowledge the support Carol and Jean provided during the writing of the book. Not to be forgotten are Colin and Megan, who shared their father with this effort and Lieutenant Savik's steadfast companionship, which lightened the lonely burden. We also wish to acknowledge those who provided us wise counsel that guided us to improving the book. Many thanks.

INTRODUCTION

In the late 1980s and early 1990s, health care has come to the forefront of the American political, economic, and social agenda. The government and employers now bear much of the cost of health care delivery and have become hard pressed to absorb the spiraling costs. Health care costs have become a major factor in balancing local, state, federal, and corporate budgets and in driving up the costs of goods and services. However, despite questions of affordability, politicians are also concerned about the growing number of people who are not receiving adequate care. Their response to the crisis of a third of our citizens having limited or no access to health care delivery is not unexpected—increased government involvement. Medicare- and Medicaid-like coverage might be considered as a way to cover all citizens, and employers might be required to provide employees a mandated baseline package of health care insurance benefits.

The health care industry's providers and insurers are also responding. Insurers, pressured by purchasers, have developed new managed care methodologies that are reducing health care costs. Physicians are lowering their costs by organizing into medical groups that reduce costly duplication of services. This reduction of duplication allows them to enter into price negotiations with managed care organizations. The response is also being led by hospital administrators who have witnessed a dramatic change in the role of their institutions in the health care delivery marketplace. The survival of these institutions now depends on the administrators adapting to new cost-conscious demands. New income-generating uses have been found for surplus beds and extra space. New ways of delivering traditional inpatient services in cost-effective outpatient settings have been developed. Hospital administrators have also realized that physicians control the utilization of their services. Meaningful physician participation in their organizations can create greater cost effectiveness, which permits hospitals to influence the health care marketplace. It is this area, the relationship between hospitals and physicians, that this book explores. More specifically the book examines the many types of synergistic relationships that hospitals can develop with physician medical groups that form large enough economic units to make affiliation meaningful and cost effective.

The Book and Its Organization

This book is organized into three sections. The first four chapters describe some of the history of the health care industry that motivates hospital administrators and physicians to move closer together. Chapters 5 through 8 discuss issues related to building these new relationships. Hospital administrators and physicians must understand the implications of these new relationships before deciding it is in their best interest to move ahead with affiliation plans. These chapters provide a framework designed to assist the reader with assessing the strategy and legality of combining their resources and their managements. In particular, Chapters 7 and 8 provide those who are not familiar with medical group practice administration a better understanding of their governance, management, and operations. Chapters 9 through 11 examine the ways that hospitals and physicians who practice in groups can bond to achieve mutual interests. These opportunities include management contracts, joint ventures, merger, and acquisition. Chapter 12 concludes the book with reflections on the pitfalls that can occur in hospital-physician relations and observations and advice on how to avoid them. This chapter also looks ahead to the future and the implications of this movement for reshaping the American health care delivery system.

Chapter 1 provides a historical overview of the growth of medical group practice and the influence this growth has had on hospitals. Statistics are provided to illustrate the rapid growth in popularity of medical groups. Also discussed is why relationships between medical groups and hospitals are of growing importance.

Chapter 2 reviews the history of physician reimbursement and how changes over the 1970s and 1980s have affected physician incomes and their relationships with hospitals and the many new managed care insurance products on the market.

Chapter 3 looks at how the major purchasers of health care have influenced the economics and practice styles of physicians. In particular the effects of these influences on physicians' use of hospital facilities is examined. The chapter points out consumers have become more sophisticated and now demand higher quality and more convenient care.

Chapter 4 examines the newest trend of hospitals and hospital corporations to create vertically integrated structures. This integration focuses on including physicians as hospitals seek to compete with other hospitals to maintain market share. This chapter introduces the theme of the remainder of the book by opening the discussion of the different ways hospitals and physicians can integrate to regain dominance in the marketplace.

Chapter 5 urges that hospital administrators and their medical staff use strategic planning as a means of achieving integration. Many hospitals fail in their attempts to win physician confidence because they cannot demonstrate that their strategic planning provides a meaningful place for physicians in their business. Expanding opportunities for physicians and hospitals to combine their efforts has also attracted the attention of Congress and state legislatures, who are cautiously watching their progress for adverse effects.

Chapter 6 reviews the legal and political concerns facing the development of new ventures. Politicians want to ensure that the public benefits from any activity that limits competition or creates potential conflicts of interest.

Chapter 7 provides an in-depth look at how medical groups govern themselves. The biggest obstacle hospital administrators have to face in successfully approaching medical groups is knowing how medical groups function. This chapter discusses how human nature, education and training, and peer pressure affect the performance of physicians as managers and leaders.

Chapter 8 provides the reader with an approach to assessing medical group operations. The chapter's content will assist those who must appraise whether medical group practices are desirable to affiliate with. The last thing hospital administrators want to do is acquire or develop an affiliation with a group practice that will require a constant flow of money and human resources to maintain.

Chapter 9 examines different approaches to affiliations. For those who want to ease into affiliations, service agreements and management contracts provide a way that each party can maintain ownership and control but enjoy some of the advantages of what the other party has to offer.

Chapter 10 deals with those groups that are ready to share ownership of their practice with a hospital in return for greater security and profit. Issues discussed include governance, management, financial arrangements, and physician responses.

Chapter 11 discusses yet another integration option. Hospitals might wish to form their own clinics and physician organizations. This becomes particularly advantageous to hospitals that service an area that is not adequately covered.

Chapter 12 concludes the book by summarizing the major themes of the book, and it warns that problems can occur if the bonding process is not handled correctly. Bonding is also examined from a public policy viewpoint. The authors speculate about how our health care system will look when hospitals have formed large integrated systems that include primary care and multispecialty medical groups.

1

THE DEVELOPMENT OF MEDICAL GROUPS: THE GROWING IMPORTANCE OF PHYSICIANS TO HOSPITALS

The practice of medicine in groups has become popular among physicians. Group practice offers physicians advantages that are explained in this chapter. Hospital administrators must appreciate why medical groups are important to doctors before launching into affiliations with them or negotiations for their management or purchase. There are also historical and statistical perspectives that are important to know. This chapter provides information that highlights the remarkable growth in the popularity of medical groups and provides some ideas on how hospitals can benefit groups. However, before beginning, we must define *medical group*.

Definition

The American Medical Association (AMA) has used the following definition of a medical group for the last 20 years. Medical group practices are defined as

> The application of medical service by three or more physicians formally organized to provide medical care, consultations, diagnosis, and/or treatment through the joint use of equipment, records, and personnel, and with income from medical practice distributed according to some prearranged plan.[1]

This definition is broad enough to encompass a variety of organizational arrangements. In particular, the definition does not rule out health maintenance organizations (HMOs) or hospital-owned medical groups as long as they remain legally separate. Affiliated medical groups must be autonomous, and an acid test of this autonomy is that a hospital or an HMO may not control physicians or pay them salaries.

Legal Organization of Medical Groups

Medical groups can take a number of different legal forms. The popularity of the different forms has changed since the 1960s. The AMA reported in 1969 that 69 percent of medical groups were partnerships, followed in popularity by professional corporations (PCs) (16 percent) and associations (9 percent).[2] However, the popularity of partnerships rapidly faded. By 1975 the PC was the most popular form of organization (61 percent). American Medical Association data for 1988 continues to show the PC to be the most popular form of organization (71 percent), followed by partnerships (16 percent) and associations (4 percent).[3] The popularity of PCs in large part is an outcome of favorable tax advantages that accrue to their members.

Numbers of Medical Groups

The numbers of medical groups expanded rapidly in the 1970s and 1980s. Figure 1.1 shows a rapid increase in number from 1969 to 1984, an increase of 143 percent (9.5 percent per year) and over 9,000 groups. The data for 1988, however, show a leveling out in the rate of increase with only a 7 percent increase or 1,100 additional groups having been formed during the late 1980s. These findings are mirrored by data on the growth in numbers of physicians practicing in groups. Between 1969 and 1984 physicians practicing in groups increased 250 percent (16.6 percent per year) to 139,127. Between 1984 and 1988 the increase was but 12 percent to 155,628. These statistics show that many physicians prefer the medical groups as a means of dealing with the realities of the marketplace and the practice of medicine. The popularity of these groups exists for a number of good reasons.

Why Medical Groups Are So Popular

There are many reasons why medical groups are a popular way to practice medicine. Some of the best reasons are discussed in the following sections.

Economies of Scale

Some of the key advantages of an organization are derived from economies of scale. For medical groups these economies include the hiring of higher-

Figure 1.1 Number of Medical Groups, 1969 to 1988

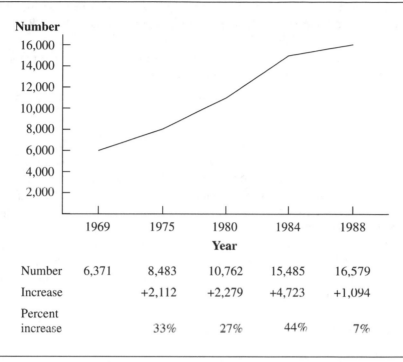

	1969	1975	1980	1984	1988
Number	6,371	8,483	10,762	15,485	16,579
Increase		+2,112	+2,279	+4,723	+1,094
Percent increase		33%	27%	44%	7%

Source: Medical Groups in the U.S. 1990 (Chicago: American Medical Association, 1990), 33.

quality staff and better use of their time. They also include better access to financing and the ability to build larger and better clinic space. They include better use of clinic equipment and the likelihood of being able to purchase and achieve optimal use of expensive diagnostic and therapeutic equipment. They include the ability to purchase and develop better communication and information systems, which enhance a group's ability to develop and maintain high-quality patient care, which is a key factor in long-term success. In sum, many of the advantages of economies of scale realized by hospitals are also realized by medical groups. Linkages with a hospital can be expected to further enhance these advantages.

Cross-Coverage and Collegiality

Physicians who practice in medical groups have colleagues with whom they can talk and discuss cases. They also gain the important advantage of having their patients covered by their colleagues when they go on trips or are ill. One last advantage is the rotation of onerous duties such as being on-call for emergencies and working evenings and weekends. Linkages with hospitals can permit the expansion of a medical group, which can further enhance these benefits, although care must be taken to not overload group members with many new hospital-based responsibilities.

Start-Up Costs

Starting a new practice can take hundreds of thousands of dollars and several years of long days and little vacation to reach a desired income level. Start-up costs and many taxing administrative difficulties have become a major factor in new physicians seeking salaried membership in medical groups. A new physician, by becoming an employee of an existing medical group, immediately overcomes the many difficulties of starting out on his or her own but with the obvious compromise of personal autonomy. The addition of a hospital to the fiscal matrix can vastly increase the potential resources available to medical groups, thereby making it easier to attract new recruits and retain valued staff.

Greater Resources and Survivability

Medical groups can develop pools of reserve financial resources and can pull their members together to deal with major problems. Both of these advantages ensure the group's survival should there be an unanticipated dip in demand for the group's services. Medical groups also have the human resources to permit them to innovate solutions to problems they encounter, such as experimenting with satellite clinics, developing new diagnostic and therapeutic services, relocating, expanding into new markets, and negotiating loans and venture capital from members or lending institutions. In sum, medical groups have human and financial resources that permit them to handle their marketing and fiscal affairs without excessive reliance on external sources. The linkage of a group to a hospital further increases resources and survivability, but at the cost of member autonomy. Hospital administrators must be sensitive to this cost to avoid letting it become too high.

Many advantages accrue to physicians who choose to join or develop medical groups. These advantages can be further enhanced if a carefully developed affiliation with a hospital is added. The following review of the frequency of various types of medical groups and their attributes further underscores their diversity and therefore the need for hospital administrators to be informed about medical groups before developing affiliations with them.

Sizes of Medical Groups

The most frequently reported size for a medical group is less than 15 members. Groups with fewer than 15 members constitute 91.4 percent of all groups responding to the AMA's survey (Table 1.1). However, Table 1.1 shows that a size in the range of 50 to 99 members has become popular, as indicated by an increase of 182 percent in the eight-year period 1980 to 1988. These findings, however, must be compared with the type of group and size of group according to the number of physicians reported as members (see the discussion below, where it is observed that despite lower numbers of large groups, they have the most members).

Medical Group Practice Types

Table 1.2 shows that single specialty groups are by far the most popular form of practice, with 11,522 groups or 71 percent reported. However, multispecialty group popularity is growing at a faster pace (20 percent growth versus 12 percent growth for single specialty), with general and family practice groups declining in number. It is noteworthy and also logical that groups with more than 25 members are most frequently multispecialty groups—those perhaps best able to support a hospital's needs. Table 1.2 also

Table 1.1 Distribution of Medical Groups by Size, 1980 to 1988

Size	1980	Percent of Total	1988	Percent of Total	Percent Increase, 1980–1988
3	3,751	34.9%	4,547	28.0%	21.2%
4	2,205	20.5	3,618	22.3	64.1
5 to 6	2,188	20.3	3,569	22.0	63.1
7 to 15	1,849	17.2	3,116	19.2	68.5
16 to 25	390	3.6	672	4.1	72.3
26 to 49	233	2.2	403	2.5	73.0
50 to 99	70	0.7	198	1.2	182.9
100+	76	0.7	118	0.7	55.3
Totals	10,762	100.0%	16,241	100.0%	50.9%

Sources: *Medical Groups in the U.S. 1980* (Chicago: American Medical Association, 1980), 15; *Medical Groups in the U.S. 1990* (Chicago: American Medical Association, 1990), 12.
Note: In 1988, there were 388 groups that did not report size.

Table 1.2 Distribution of Medical Groups by Type of Practice and Size, 1984 to 1988

Size	Single Specialty			Multispecialty			Family Practice			Totals		
	1984	1988	Percent Increase	1984	1988	Percent Increase	1984	1988	Percent Increase	1984	1988	Percent Increase
3	3,622	3,460	-4.5%	408	446	9.3%	723	641	-11.3%	4,753	4,547	-4.3%
4	2,497	2,775	11.1	297	413	39.1	454	430	-5.3	3,248	3,618	11.4
5 to 6	2,212	2,702	22.2	392	572	45.9	314	295	-6.1	2,918	3,569	22.3
7 to 15	1,584	2,109	33.1	768	843	9.8	149	164	10.1	2,501	3,116	24.6
16 to 25	210	326	55.2	265	307	15.8	40	39	-2.5	515	672	30.5
26 to 49	85	103	21.2	242	286	18.2	25	14	-44.0	352	403	14.5
50 to 99	38	37	-2.6	106	161	51.9	4	0	-100.0	148	198	33.8
100+	19	10	-47.4	132	107	-18.9	3	1	-66.7	154	118	-23.4
Total	10,267	11,522	12.2%	2,610	3,135	20.1%	1,712	1,584	-7.5%	14,589	16,241	11.3%

Sources: Medical Groups in the U.S. 1984 (Chicago: American Medical Association, 1984), 26; *Medical Groups in the U.S. 1990* (Chicago: American Medical Association, 1990), 12.

Note: In 1990, there were 254 groups with unknown size and 84 with unknown size and specialty.

shows a clear trend in size preference for single, general, and family practice groups, with groups with 7 to 25 members being the most preferred.

Distribution of Physicians by Type of Group

Table 1.3 provides a slightly different look at the most popular types of groups and sizes. The findings remain similar to those of Table 1.2; however, multispecialty groups become the dominant influence, reporting 49 percent of all physicians as compared to 46 percent for single specialty and 5 percent for general and family practice. It is particularly important to note that there are 36,414 physicians reported in medical groups with more than 100 members, 22 percent of all physicians in medical groups, whereas in Table 1.2 multispecialty groups with more than 100 members constituted less than 1 percent of the groups reported.

Frequency of Type of Hospital Affiliation

Table 1.4 shows the popularity of different types of hospital affiliations. One percent (1.05 percent) of medical groups are owned and operated by a hospital where the hospital assumes fiscal responsibility for the group and pays the physicians. An additional 1 percent (0.92 percent) are owned by an organization that also owns one or more hospitals. A little more than 3 percent (3.44 percent) of the groups reported they were associated with a hospital where the hospital assumed joint fiscal responsibility for the group, including physician compensation. It is noteworthy that physician bonding through landlord arrangements accounts for almost 10 percent of the affiliations (9.68 percent). By far the most popular type of affiliation is for group members to have hospital privileges. Seventy-four percent (73.59 percent) of the groups reported this type of arrangement. It is readily concluded that hospital ownership and direct participation in medical groups' fiscal affairs accounts for little more than 5 percent of all the different types of affiliation arrangements. That means that the expansion of hospitals into the ownership and operation of medical groups is a new phenomenon that will require the management of new uncertainties and risks that cannot be minimized until there is greater industrywide experience.

Distribution of Medical Groups by Specialty and Size

Table 1.5 provides information about the relative sizes of medical groups by medical specialty. The table is arranged from lowest frequency to highest

Table 1.3 Distribution of Medical Group Physicians by Type of Practice and Size, 1984 to 1988

Size	Single Specialty			Multispecialty			General or Family Practice			Totals		
	1984	1988	Percent Increase	1984	1988	Percent Increase	1984	1988	Percent Increase	1984	1988	Percent Increase
3	10,787	10,380	−3.8%	1,196	1,338	11.9%	2,142	1,923	−10.2%	14,125	13,641	−3.4%
4	9,988	11,100	11.1	1,188	1,652	39.1	1,816	1,720	−5.3	12,992	14,472	11.4
5 to 6	11,833	14,473	22.3	2,138	3,103	45.1	1,665	1,590	−4.5	15,636	19,166	22.6
7 to 15	14,571	19,650	34.9	7,658	8,370	9.3	1,360	1,463	7.6	23,589	29,483	25.0
16 to 25	4,099	6,254	52.6	5,306	6,052	14.1	803	803	0.0	10,208	13,109	28.4
26 to 49	2,812	3,435	22.2	8,370	10,029	19.8	790	408	−48.4	11,972	13,872	15.9
50 to 99	2,481	2,330	−6.1	7,101	10,952	54.2	246	0	−100.0	9,828	13,282	35.1
100 +	3,346	4,239	26.7	36,414	34,264	−5.9	1,017	100	−90.2	40,777	38,603	−5.3
Total	59,917	71,861	19.9%	69,371	75,760	9.2%	9,839	8,007	−18.6%	139,127	155,628	11.9%

Source: Medical Groups in the U.S. 1984 (Chicago: American Medical Association, 1984), 27; *Medical Groups in the U.S. 1990* (Chicago: American Medical Association, 1990), 12.

Table 1.4   Frequency of Type of Hospital Affiliation, 1988

Hospital Affiliation	Size of Medical Groups Reported					
	3 to 9	*10 to 25*	*26 to 49*	*>50*	*Total*	*Percent*
Hospital and group owned by same entity	33	32	5	19	89	0.92%
Hospital owns and operates group	68	24	4	5	101	1.05
Hospital associated	233	71	15	12	331	3.44
Hospital is landlord	756	116	38	22	932	9.68
Hospital privileges	6,200	647	142	95	7,084	73.59
Group provides services	444	125	16	9	594	6.17
Other affiliation	156	47	8	15	226	2.35
No affiliation	236	21	9	3	269	2.79
Total	8,126	1,083	237	180	9,626	100.00%

Source: *Medical Groups in the U.S. 1990* (Chicago: American Medical Association, 1990), 23.

frequency. Seven specialties (cardiovascular diseases, general surgery, neurology, ophthalmology, orthopedics, pathology, and psychiatry) have the fewest physicians in groups. They, in all cases, individually represent less than 5 percent and together only 24 percent of all physicians reported. The small sizes of these specialty groups can be explained as the result of their highly specialized types of practice; some are also faced with other health care delivery competitors as is the case in ophthalmology (optometrists) and psychiatry (social workers).

Five specialties (anesthesiology, emergency medicine, obstetrics and gynecology (OB/GYN), pediatrics, and radiology) have substantially more physicians practicing in groups (with the exception of OB/GYN, 10,000 or more). They represent a midrange in size and account for 38 percent of all physicians reported to be practicing in groups. It is noteworthy that emergency medicine is a new specialization and already represents a significant number of physicians in medical groups. Greater competition and increasing indigent care are forcing medical groups to greater responsiveness to a broader range of urgent or emergency health care problems.

Those physicians most often practicing in groups are family and general medicine (17,302, 12 percent), internal medicine (21,343, 14 percent), and all others (17,639, 12 percent). The traditional gatekeepers of the health care system—family, general, and internal medicine physicians—represent the largest numbers of physicians practicing in medical groups.

Table 1.5   Distribution of Medical Groups by Specialty and Size, 1988

	Number	*Percent of Total*
0 to 5 percent		
Cardiovascular diseases	5,241	4%
General surgery	7,165	5
Neurology	2,674	2
Ophthalmology	3,886	3
Orthopedic surgery	6,628	4
Pathology	5,072	3
Psychiatry	4,891	3
Subtotal	35,557	24%
6 to 10 percent		
Anesthesiology	10,052	7%
Emergency medicine	11,461	8
OB/GYN	9,390	6
Pediatrics	11,509	8
Radiology	14,009	9
Subtotal	56,421	38%
> 11 percent		
Family/general medicine	17,302	12%
Internal medicine	21,343	14
Other	17,639	12
Subtotal	56,284	38%
Total	148,262	100%

Source: *Medical Groups in the U.S. 1990* (Chicago: American Medical Association, 1990), 35.

Additional Highlights

The AMA concluded their 1990 report on medical groups by making a number of noteworthy predictions.[4]

- The number of medical groups will continue to increase; however, there will also be an increased rate of merger and dissolution as groups respond to the changing marketplace and their financial constraints. Mergers can be expected to result in ever larger groups that account for an ever greater percentage of physicians practicing in groups. Hospital administrators can also have an active role in merging their institutions with medical groups to create marketplace competitors of truly significant proportions.

- Managed care (HMOs and preferred provider organizations [PPOs]) will serve as a force that encourages the growth of medical groups as health care delivery is shifted from hospitals to ambulatory settings. In particular, the AMA notes that hospitals must diversify and must bond or bind the providers of ambulatory services to their institutions. Purchase, merger, and the management of groups is a direct route to achieving this desired goal.

- Medical groups that are able to demonstrate to the public and others that they deliver quality-assured services while maintaining cost effectiveness will be assured of success. Hospital administrators are in especially good positions to help medical groups develop and maintain quality-assured and cost-effective operations that will reduce the risk of linking with medical groups.

- Larger groups will be most successful, as they have the financial and human resources to support the constant expansion of services and service modalities. Larger groups can also support better staff recruitment and the development of much needed computerized information systems. Hospital administrators are in an excellent position to further enhance the benefits of these trends and can, in many instances, make it possible for groups to offer even more services than they ever contemplated.

- Medical groups will become more geographically dispersed and more specialized in local markets. These trends point to diversification and the development of marketing niches as survival strategies. Hospital administrators can actively help groups to develop and implement strategic plans that can become more aggressive when a hospital's financial, information, and human resources are available to support this work.

- Last, the AMA predicts the economic interests of hospitals and groups will drive them closer together through such mechanisms as hospital ownership, multiple cooperation agreements, management contracts, and joint ventures.

Conclusion

Medical groups have become an important factor in the health care delivery marketplace and offer hospital administrators many opportunities to expand their market share by bonding and even binding medical groups to them through a variety of mechanisms. Medical groups represent a new frontier for hospital administrators to learn about and to enter into. The balance of this book is devoted to informing hospital administrators about medical groups and the many ways hospitals and groups can benefit from affiliating with each other.

Notes

1. P. Havlicek, *Medical Groups in the U.S. 1990* (Chicago: American Medical Association, 1990), 5.
2. Ibid., 36.
3. Ibid., 36.
4. Ibid., 37–39.

2

THE EVOLUTION OF THE ECONOMICS OF MEDICAL PRACTICE

There are many reasons why physicians and hospitals should work more closely together, the biggest being economics. Government and industry cost-containment measures have forced health care providers to lower their costs to keep health care affordable. The diagnostic-related group (DRG) methodology, combined with managed care initiatives, has attempted to contain hospital costs by making providers financially responsible for both the efficacy of and the costs of services rendered. The 1990s will see Medicare implement the resource-based relative value system (RBRVS), which continues this trend for physicians. This system promises to contain costs and redistribute reimbursement between medical specialties. Private insurance companies are expected to follow suit and make the overall impact of RBRVS on medical practices dramatic.

There are also adverse changes occurring on the cost side of the physician's income statement. Physicians are hiring more staff to respond to patient demands and to handle paperwork associated with managed care plans and Medicare. Another example of an expense that continues to rise is professional liability insurance, which has had a major impact on surgeons and obstetricians.

These economic trends have cut into physician income. Physicians must work harder to negate the effects of these trends or else be continually dissatisfied with their bottom line. This chapter examines the evolution of the financial aspects of practicing medicine, an evolution that is irresistibly moving the interests of physicians and hospitals closer together.

Changes in Reimbursement to Physicians

Physicians have been obliged to accept a steady decrease in their power in the marketplace as changes in reimbursement policies by major third party payers have come to dominate health care financing. The effects of these changes can be understood from several different vantage points.

Fee-for-Service Payment

Physicians have traditionally enjoyed tremendous control over their income. The fee-for-service (FFS) payment methodology meant that physicians could charge and be reimbursed for any amount they desired, with the exception that they could not discriminate in their charges by payer. There were no controls over their fee setting. The only factor they considered in setting fees was what other physicians in their specialty were charging. Fees were set not so much for the purpose of competition but to not look out of line in the eyes of other physicians. The only exception was when they perceived that their skills were better by comparison. Doctor Smith might, for example, have kept his fee schedule 5 percent higher than Doctor Jones based on his belief that his skills were marginally better. In sum, physicians did not have to contend with a marketplace function that regulated their fees. They merely set their fees to achieve a desired income. A 10 percent increase in income meant a 10 percent increase in fees, assuming volume remained the same.

Fixed Fee Payment Schedules

The FFS approach to provider reimbursement had one major flaw: it did not limit the costs of health care for those paying for it. During the 1970s and 1980s major third party payers and employers decided that they needed more control over their costs. Physician costs had to be regulated. However, rather than dictating what physicians could charge, one approach that they used was to reimburse physicians based on the average fees submitted by all physicians in a specialty within established geographic regions of the country. This approach marked the first attempt by the government (Medicare and Medicaid) and the private insurance industry, through associations like the Health Insurance Association of America (HIAA), to use fixed fee payment schedules.

In addition to establishing a fixed maximum limit, the methodology was expanded to include the "lesser of" policy where the payer reimbursed at the fixed rate or the actual fee, whichever was less. Fixed payment schedules had the effect of lowering reimbursement to physicians who charged too much while continuing to pay those that charged less than the limits the lower rates they requested.

This initial attempt at cost containment gradually became focused on adjusting the percent of the mean to be reimbursed. This usually translated into ever increasing contractual adjustments and larger amounts being collected from patients in those cases in which contractual adjustments were not obligatory. It also meant that increasing fees did not readily translate into increased income. If a physician's fee schedule exceeded the payer's fixed amount, increased fees often only meant increased contractual adjustments when the assignment of benefits was accepted.

However, the fixed payment schedule methodology also had its limitations. Insurance companies and health plans needed good actuarial experience to develop the reimbursement schedules, data that were not always available. Another limitation was that the schedules had to be accepted by physicians. They had to agree to accept the payment reimbursement schedules as payment in full. In most instances physicians did not find the amount reimbursed to be acceptable and billed the patient for the difference. Although in some areas of the country, where physicians found themselves competing with one another for patients covered by Medicare, Blue Cross Blue Shield, HMOs, and insurance companies, physicians often found that they had little choice but to participate. Nonetheless, these limitations led the industry to explore new reimbursement methodologies.

Risk Sharing: Capitation and Payment Reserves

Managed care introduced a new approach to reimbursing participating primary care physicians. Actuaries computed the average cost per person per year and allocated participating providers this amount as a budget for primary care providers for health plan enrollees. The money awarded is fixed and assumed variations in the intensity of services are averaged out. This assumption created risk. If an individual or group of primary care physicians encountered costs that exceeded the capitation budget, they assumed some responsibility for paying for the overage out of their own pockets. As a result, primary care physicians, who were contractually liable for thousands of enrollees, assumed the risks for paying other physicians and hospitals for some of their cost overruns.

Another form of risk sharing that evolved was the reserve payment method. This method enabled managed care plans to extend risk sharing to specialty physicians, who are not in a gatekeeper role. In this scheme, a portion of the agreed-to FFS payment is held by the payer until year end. These reserve withholding risk pools constitute anywhere from 15 to 25 percent of the approved payment. To avoid this outcome, participating physicians are guided by utilization criteria that they are expected to meet for their panel of patients. Typical cost-containment criteria include

- the cost of physician services per patient per year,
- the number of visits per patient per year, and
- the amount of ancillary services per patient per year.

If these cost-containment criteria are met, the reserve pool is released to the physician at the end of the year. If the criteria are not met or only partially met, part or all of the risk pool withheld is maintained by the plan, and the physician has to write off the loss. A 20 percent unpaid withholding could, for example, lower a physician's reimbursement to 50 percent of his or her original charge.

Resource-Based Relative Value System

None of the previous methodologies have been entirely effective in lowering physician costs. With the development of RBRVS, the government and health insurers hope they have found the method that will do the job. The architects of this new payment scheme have attempted to put a value on the services provided by physicians based on how much time, effort, and resources are involved in delivering the service. This system is a big departure from the other attempts at cost containment because it defines the market price for a physician's service rather than trying to discount fees set by physicians.

It is believed that RBRVS will accomplish several goals. It will promote primary care specialties and case management and base payments on average physician work and expense and not on the specialty of the physician. Surgeons and procedure-oriented specialties are predicted to see the largest reimbursement reductions under this new method of payment. The feared impact of RBRVS is that the shifts in payments might encourage physicians to discontinue serving Medicare beneficiaries. However, if this happens, many states appear to be ready to force physicians to participate in Medicare as a condition of licensure.

In sum, the implementation of RBRVS is yet another step along the path of containing costs by limiting physician reimbursement. This system is expected to reduce income and tighten cash flows for physicians during times when practice costs are rising. The following sections examine the other side of the equation: the factors contributing to the upward spiral of practice costs.

The Rising Cost of Medical Practice

Physicians and their business managers are faced with declining reimbursement and increasing operating costs. Many factors are contributing to increasing the cost of medical practice. The most significant are as follows:

- Managed care plans have required physicians to increase the size of their nonphysician staff to perform compliance and paperwork tasks.
- Advances in health care technology and competition have increased the consumption of ancillary services in physician offices. Radiology, laboratory, physical therapy, and medical-surgical supplies are commonly provided.
- Increased professional liability threats have inflated malpractice insurance premiums.
- Increasing patient demand and a shift to providing outpatient care have required physicians to expand their facilities and staffs.
- Physician groups must guarantee new physicians' salaries at increasingly competitive amounts.

Third Party Payer Demands That
Increase Office Operating Expenses

Medical practice operating expenses have increased for two reasons. Managed care programs have imposed time-consuming and costly requirements on where and how physician services are to be delivered, and they have increased the complexity of the paperwork for claims processing. Health maintenance organizations and PPOs have restructured the delivery of health care by physicians. Primary care physicians who accept risk-sharing contracts have had to adopt resource-consuming strategies to manage the consumption of service while trying to maintain quality and meet patient health care expectations.

Increasing patient care demands and efficiency considerations have also limited the time physicians have to oversee the administration of managed care contracts. The solution has been to hire additional office staff to process referral authorizations and claims, make appointments with specialists, call in and report hospital admissions, and handle plan quality assurance and utilization review requirements. Plans that have special contractual arrangements with certain hospitals, medical equipment vendors, pharmacies, or mental health specialists can make proper handling of patient health care needs a bureaucratic nightmare. Although patients are supposed to be responsible for knowing and following their plan's procedures, it is often the physician who is caught in the middle. Referring errors lead to unhappy patients when they become responsible for paying the costs out their own pockets. The complexity is further aggravated by frequent changes in the features and procedures of health plans, which make it difficult for enrollees and physicians to know which services are covered and which become the responsibility of the patient. These factors have forced physicians to be responsible for knowing both patients' coverage and their plans' rules and procedures. If a patient's plan has a copayment, deductible, or noncovered service, the physicians must know. The volume and complexity of claims processing and reporting has also required many physician offices to use costly computer systems to manage these functions. These systems then often become difficult and expensive to operate and often require the hiring of new staff with the expertise to manage them.

Increasing Consumption and Practice Costs

Patients are utilizing more services. Increased technology, managed care, preventive care, and a better knowledge of what is available have combined to increase consumption.

Increased technology. Vastly improved technology has encouraged utilization. Physicians who wish to leave no stone unturned to ensure proper diagnosis and treatment are consuming more radiology and laboratory testing, which are being reimbursed at ever lower rates. Tightened profit margins have led physicians to use break-even analysis to decide whether to continue or expand in-office radiology and laboratory testing. At the same time, physicians often feel that they are being pressured to overutilize diagnostic testing to cover themselves from the threat of malpractice lawsuits.

Managed care. Managed care plans that provide complete coverage and have low copayments create demand as enrollees feel that they should take advantage of this "free" care and see their physicians when they want to. These trends have increased pressure on the scheduling and gatekeeping responsibilities of primary care physicians.

Preventive care. Preventive care is slowly taking hold with health plans and physicians. Unfortunately, these services are still not cost effective for physicians to offer because third party payers are not, as yet, providing enough reimbursement. However, conscientious physicians often absorb the cost of these services because it is good medicine.

Informed patients. Gatekeeping physicians are now more often confronted with informed but costly patient demands that cannot always be resisted. Better consumer knowledge of available services and better understanding of health care issues have combined to make consumers much more interested and even aggressive about seeking services. Efforts by the government and nonprofit groups to alert the public to the dangers of cancer, heart disease, and other life-threatening illnesses have motivated people to monitor their health status more. Cholesterol level tests, blood pressure monitoring, and cancer screening procedures have become popular requests of patients.

The rising cost of malpractice. One of the more publicized expense increases that physicians are facing is the rising cost for professional liability insurance. Larger numbers of law suits as well as higher attorney fees and awards have driven up premiums. The hardest hit specialties have been OB/GYN and surgeons of all types.

Space. The shift to outpatient care has increased demand for clinic office space. Real estate prices have steadily escalated, making doctor office rent expensive. The cost of developing one's own space has also become prohibitive due to the amount of capital needed to furnish and equip a modern physician's office.

The cost of recruiting and retaining new physicians. Physicians who are looking for practice opportunities are seeing their worth as a provider escalating while the economic advantages of being an owner of a medical practice are waning. Geographic and absolute shortages of physicians in some specialties have driven up the costs groups and hospitals must absorb to land an available physician. Recruitment is made all the more difficult by physician willingness to accept employment in nontraditional practice situations ranging from staffing HMO clinics and hospital emergency rooms to temporary locum tenens in exciting parts of the country.

This type of competition has made it expensive and difficult for physician groups to add to their ranks. Expensive recruitment packages must be assembled that include salary guarantees, bonuses, relocation expenses, insurance coverage, generous vacation benefits, and continuing education allowances. Additionally, with the increase in the number of women going into medicine, new benefits are being offered such as extended parenting leave and less weekend and evening call.

In sum, physician income is going down while operating costs are rising. These adverse economics of medical practice are leading many physicians to reconsider the benefits of independent private practice, and they are beginning to consider what hospitals might have to offer them.

What Hospitals Have That Physicians Need

Physicians, who are faced with uncertain and hard-to-understand financial futures, are approaching hospital administrators for help. Given the historically complex and all too often adversarial relationship between hospital administrators and the members of their medical staff, one might find it unusual that physicians are seeking assistance from hospitals. However, one need not look too far to see why physicians are changing their attitudes toward hospital administrators.

A number of financial and business management considerations are encouraging physicians to look for outside help. Physicians are finding that medical group practices are big, hard-to-run businesses, and they have turned to professional managers to help them run their practices. Despite better management, there is a growing number of medical groups that are financially marginal, whether they be primary care groups in high-risk capitation arrangements, groups with poor billing and collection procedures, or groups with large debts or unfundable capital expenditure needs.

Financial instability and difficulty in structuring capital have created situations with limited options. Physicians who have set themselves up as for-profit sole proprietorships or PCs are required to pay corporate taxes. If corporate taxes are higher than for personal income, the physician is encouraged to remove all net income from the practice. This incentive to withdraw earnings discourages the formation of capital through retained earnings, and borrowing becomes the only means to raise capital for large expenditures such as paying off a large HMO risk liability or financing a new physician recruit. However, borrowing can be difficult. In this day and age of bank and savings and loan failures and corporate bankruptcy, lenders are very careful about who they loan money to. Bankers often have trouble dealing with loan requests from physician corporations because practice income often goes right to the physician's pocket. The only practice asset that appeals to bankers are accounts receivable, which must be heavily discounted, and this situation leads lenders to request that the physicians personally guarantee loans.

Hospitals, on the other hand, have both the legal structure and financial wherewithal to provide capital for medical groups. As nonprofit entities, many hospitals are allowed to accumulate reserves up to a point. What better use of these reserves than to develop or strengthen medical groups that will admit their patients to the hospital. However, this might not be as straightforward as it seems. If a medical group's financial request is the result of inadequate cash flow due to poor business performance, the hospital might want to protect its investment by asking some of its management staff to consult to the practice to improve its operations. Taking this step forges a new linkage where hospital management expertise can be brought to bear and lead to a formal business partnership.

At the same time, physicians are beginning to realize that times have changed and that it is no longer reasonable to deal with hospital administrators from the traditional adversarial position. They are beginning to appreciate that hospitals are often the cornerstone for local, regional, or even national health care delivery. Physicians are also beginning to look for new bonding opportunities that benefit both parties and will ensure the financial stability they need to practice medicine.

The joining of physicians with hospitals also promises other advantages. For example, the larger economic unit promises to create a countervailing force to the economic and political force posed by managed health plans and large employers who are struggling to control health care utilization through cost containment. Hospital financial clout can translate into other advantages for medical groups. One example is simply being able to join a managed care plan. For example, primary care physicians might be able to structure their capitation arrangement to include their hospital sharing in some or most of the risk, an arrangement that shields the group from unexpected losses that would otherwise preclude their involvement. Chapter 4 will continue the discussion of the advantages.

There are also personal reasons that hospital outreach directors cite about why physicians are approaching hospitals for financial help. Physicians in small groups fear the future. The health care milieu is moving so fast for some that they fear being overcome in its big business posture. Yet another reason is older physicians, whose retirement equity is contingent on the sale of their practice and who are looking to hospitals to repay them for their years of medical staff loyalty by buying or arranging for the sale of their practices—which can be an important source of hospital admissions.

What Physicians Have That Hospitals Need

The promise of a new era in hospital-physician relations has not arisen solely because medical groups are financially troubled. This change has also been fueled by the realization by hospital administrators that successful hospitals need successful physicians on their medical staffs.

Hospitals initially tried to go it alone. Competition forced many hospitals to advertise in newspapers and on radio and television to market their services. Maternity care, chemical dependency treatment, nutrition and dietetics, outpatient physical therapy, and radiology are examples of services hospitals have marketed directly to the public. However, after spending great sums of money on this approach, hospital administrators have realized that the public is not as self-directed in seeking services as they thought. Although there might be a new sense of patient consumerism, physicians are the gatekeepers who decide what services their patients will consume and often where. Hospitals, to be successful, must recruit and then retain physicians on their staffs. Bonding with medical groups to make them larger and more successful promises to be a win-win situation for all concerned.

In sum, hospital administrators are learning that standing by and watching the demise of influential medical groups is self-defeating. Bailing out affiliated medical groups has become a necessary investment for hospitals to protect their market share and to keep competing hospitals from coming in to rescue a group and changing their referral pattern. Hospital administrators are also realizing how important the physicians are to the institution in its delivery of care. Quality assurance and patient case management, demanded by third party payers, are primarily directed by physicians. Physicians are also assuming greater responsibilities for the day-to-day and strategic management of hospitals than they had ten years ago.

Conclusion

Physicians have passed through tumultuous financial times during the past ten years. The payers for health care services have progressively tightened up the level of payments to physicians while practice costs have continued to rise. These financial stresses are gradually forcing physicians to look to hospitals and hospitals to look to physicians to enhance their collective financial survival.

3

THE HEALTH CARE MARKET AND THE CONTROL OF HEALTH CARE DELIVERY

Much has changed about the practice of medicine. Prior to the 1960s, physicians and hospitals were exempt from financial and regulatory control because they symbolized caring and healing. Physicians were healers, and hospitals were a place where the sick and injured were treated and convalesced back to health. The art of healing and saving lives was sacred, and the issue of cost was of secondary importance.

Since the 1960s, health care delivery has passed through a major transformation to become a large, complex industry absorbing close to 15 percent of the gross national product. Health care costs and demand have dramatically skyrocketed. The costs of qualified staff have grown rapidly, as have the costs of facilities and technology. The new administrative bureaucracy and the industry now see the public, not as patients, but as consumers of services who expect services to be subjected to utilization review and quality assurance to ensure low costs and high quality.

Chapter 2 discussed the history of and questionable success of efforts to contain costs through reimbursement reform. This chapter continues the discussion of cost containment by examining it as a struggle for control over patient care decision making.

The Struggle for Control

It is generally recognized today that uncontrollable costs in the health care industry have become an economic problem for individuals, employers, and the government. As a result, cost containment has come to mean more than

27

just keeping costs down. The control of costs has become a struggle for the control of the patient care decision-making process.

In the "golden era" of medicine, physicians delivered health care without much consideration to its costs. The public accepted physician decisions, and responsible third parties paid for them. Today, attitudes have changed in that insurance companies, employers, and the public want to be involved in the decision-making process of health care delivery. Individuals want control over their care and lives, and third party payers, employers, and the government want to be assured that quality care is delivered at a low price.

As a result, the struggle for cost control is pitting providers against payers, and hospital administrators and physicians are beginning to realize that they are on the same side in the control issue. They are beginning to look to each other as they now jointly ask the question, How do we maintain the control of our industry?

Many factors are contributing to the struggle for control. Four of the most significant issues are

1. the creation of powerful managed care delivery systems—HMOs and PPOs,
2. the development of interest by employers in reducing costs while improving the quality of the health care their employees receive,
3. advances in technology that have altered the delivery of care and created an interdisciplinary struggle for the control of the technology, and
4. changes in the attitudes of patients as consumers.

These issues have had a major impact on changing the marketplace milieu that the health care delivery system operates in.

The Creation of Alternative Delivery Systems: Managed Care

Managed care is a driving force that has altered the health care delivery system. In the past, patients sought care on their own using whichever physician they felt could meet their needs and, once selected, the physician was in complete control of what services were to be provided and where. Hospitals fulfilled the role of being the place where physicians brought their patients to receive services.

The system worked well for many years; however, as costs escalated, the government, insurance companies, and employers realized that they were at the mercy of the providers and had little or no input into what the providers were doing. A new system was needed that provided new cost-conscious motivations for how and why care was delivered. Although different health care delivery models surfaced, the HMO emerged as the new cost-conscious managed care approach.

Managed Care: The Health Maintenance Organization

The notion of managed care arose with the introduction of HMOs. Health maintenance organizations were originally designed to promote health maintenance and illness prevention. Rather than being a system of restorative health care delivery that dealt with illness and injury, the notion was to use a model that encouraged patients to utilize physicians and other health professionals to maintain good health. Examples included structured prenatal care, well-child examinations and immunizations, breast cancer screening, nutrition and dietetics counseling, and family planning. The model assumed patient and doctor would work together to make the right choices. Payers hoped that this shared decision-making process would contain costs.

Health maintenance organization plans were easy to sell to employers and the government. Shared patient-doctor decision making was to cut down on the delivery of marginal services, which, it was believed, were the result of an uninformed public, overprescribing physicians, and the practice of defensive medicine. Financial reward structures of HMOs contributed to controlling the cost by creating reimbursement methodologies that encouraged physicians to make more cost-effective decisions that suppressed the total consumption of services. Physicians and, to a lesser extent, patients were coerced into the role of gatekeepers and made to feel responsible for the total consumption of services. As a result, the control of the payment mechanism by HMOs led to them sharing in decision making in health care delivery with patients, physicians, and hospitals.

The Gatekeeper System

The development of managed care delivery systems marked a transition from a free market to one where control and rationing was the norm. Enrollees in HMOs could no longer roam the medical marketplace picking and choosing the type of physician and services they felt they needed. Specialists and emergency rooms could no longer serve as an enrollee's primary source of care. Primary care physicians became the gatekeepers and assumed a new position of power relative to both hospitals and their colleagues the specialty physicians because of their new decision-making authority over health care delivery. Enrollees in HMO plans were required to identify a primary care physician who would then manage their health care needs including authorizing everything from prescriptions to referrals to specialist physicians and hospitals.

To make matters worse, HMO cost-containment incentives and risk-sharing methodologies ultimately forced primary care physicians to shop around for services at the best price. The shopping focused on locating the most cost-effective providers of the more expensive services: inpatient hospital care, specialty consultation, outpatient surgery, and advanced diagnostic services. In larger markets, shopping gave the primary care physician an incentive to locate hospitals willing to offer discounted costs or to assume some of the cost risks in return for admissions.

In sum, managed care has forced enrollees and nongatekeeper providers to subordinate their interests to those of the primary care physicians. Primary care physician groups now control millions of health care consumers. Specialty referral physicians, hospitals, mental health providers, and a variety of other health care professionals who support primary care physicians in the management of their patients have been forced to cater to this new structure of health care decision making. The independence of selection by patients, primary care physicians, hospitals, and specialists has been rapidly eliminated.

Preferred Provider Organizations

Soon after the arrival of HMOs, a less restrictive form of managed care, the PPO, was developed. Preferred provider organizations tackled the issue of cost containment by negotiating volume discounts with a limited number of hospitals and physicians and then encouraging patients to choose from among them or else pay a higher cost. This approach channels patients to providers while guaranteeing enrollees greater freedom of choice than an HMO.

In sum, while HMOs use primary care physicians as the core of their provider network, PPOs are built primarily around a core of hospital participants that have staff physicians who are expected to join the PPO.

The impact of PPOs on physicians and hospitals has been significant. Preferred provider networks lead to competition among hospitals that must discount their services to be included in the network. Presumably the most cost-competitive hospitals win out in the bidding process. Physicians on the medical staff of a nonparticipating hospital must then not participate, change, or add an affiliation to a hospital that has been selected to participate to avoid seeing their patients forced to go to another physician who has admitting privileges to a participating hospital. This is a real risk for a physician group that has a large number of patients who have their health insurance plan changed to a PPO that their affiliated hospital is not a member of. Should this occur, the physician group is forced to use a participating hospital and, possibly, establish another office on or near the campus of the participating hospital.

Competition between hospitals for participating status in local PPOs has also led hospitals to create their own PPOs to maintain market share and possibly reap some profits. Preferred provider organizations are less regulated than HMOs, thus making them easier to establish and operate. Preferred provider organizations are relatively easy to market through insurance brokers who sell plans of all sorts to employer groups. Hospitals, by creating their own PPOs, also hope to bond their medical staffs and maintain their market share, thus preventing the shifting of some physician groups to other hospitals who are participating in a competing PPO. Preferred provider organizations are also gaining in popularity with employers because they can see cost savings and hear fewer complaints from their employees than was the case with physician gatekeepers.

Recapitulation

The struggle for the control of decision making in health care delivery with HMOs and PPOs is apparent. Health maintenance organizations, while leaving physicians in charge of clinical decision making, restrict the scope of what they can consider by forcing them to be cost conscious, which leads to rationing. Physicians are also limited by whom or where they can refer patients to as they may have become responsible for negotiating with other physicians and hospitals to achieve lower costs. Preferred provider organizations use hospitals as the core of their provider network. This arrangement causes them and physicians to jockey for a preferred position relative to their peers.

Participation in an HMO or a PPO of any significant size is a crucial event for both hospitals and physicians. The market penetration of managed care plans is approaching 50 percent in many cities and states, and it is getting more difficult for providers to be able not to participate without suffering significant financial consequences. However, participation often requires physicians to move or establish new offices to get into a desired plan. But mobility has its costs both financially and in the logistical problems associated with a practice that is spread out all over town. One might conclude that it is in the best interest of hospitals and physicians to work together to maintain some control of HMOs and PPOs so they are not permitted to use economics as the principal driver of medical decision making.

Employer Influences in the Health Care Marketplace

When asked, most employers will say that the rising cost of providing medical insurance for their employees is one of their biggest problems. Most employers want to provide their employees with health insurance coverage; however, the reality is that the high cost and tougher economic times make it difficult to do. As a result, employers are looking to the managed care movement to give them cost-effective choices to offer to their employees.

Employers usually have two objectives in selecting a health insurance plan. The first is to provide employees with a provider network that offers both quality and cost-effective health care. The second objective is to tailor an affordable benefit package that meets the needs of their employees. These objectives have led employers to contracting with or developing HMOs and PPOs, which has created a struggle for the control of these types of health care plans between the employer and its employees.

Employers are becoming interested in identifying high quality and cost-effective health care providers to send their employees to. These efforts have led to direct contracting between employers and health care providers—hospitals, physicians, mental health and chemical dependency centers, physical rehabilitation and chiropractors—for services ranging from prenatal care to job-related injuries and injury prevention. Contracting has occurred at all levels of care, both locally and nationally. Small companies have identified local primary care groups and hospitals for employees who live and work near the providers. Large companies with employees at locations all over the country have tapped into national health care networks that provide tertiary care services such as organ transplantation, burn care, and spinal cord injury treatment. Large numbers of employees increase the potential need for these types of services to the point that it is worthwhile to contract for them.

Direct contracting has also led employers to deal directly with providers on the cost of their services. Employers with large numbers of employees are in a position to bargain the costs down. A trend that further encourages this practice is self-insurance. Self-insuring has become a popular way to fund health benefit programs because it eliminates costs that insurance companies pass along to the employers. Marketing and administrative costs, risk insurance, and, most importantly, profits all stay in the pockets of the employer if the work and financial risk can be absorbed. Self-insurers often fine-tune their programs by contracting with a health plan to maintain enrollee information, utilization data, claims processing, and provider contracting.

Employers are also influencing their health insurance costs by shaping benefit packages to meet the specific needs of their employees. Benefit administrators have found that increasing competition between health insurers opened up this opportunity to design their own benefit packages. For example, some employers have found that the standard mental health and chemical dependency benefits exceed the needs of their employees and result in overpurchasing. By the same token, some businesses are stressful places to work in and increase the incidence of drug and alcohol abuse thereby making the need for treatment and counseling an important benefit. Highly structured prenatal care programs have also been found to have an impact on the absenteeism of pregnant employees.

In sum, employers are beginning to take charge of their health care costs and have become a major new player in the health care delivery arena. The resulting struggle for cost and quality control has put hospitals and physicians in the new position of having to demonstrate their quality and cost effectiveness to employers, not to mention having to negotiate and compete for service contracts. Hospitals and their affiliated physicians are virtually obligated to work together to deal with employers who want to purchase health care services in much the same way as they purchase the materials that go into the production of the products they sell. In communities where there is an oversupply of hospitals or physicians, this purchasing pressure is forcing providers either to deal or to lose market share.

Technological Advances in Medicine

Every year there are new and improved high-technology ways to diagnose and treat diseases. This explosion of technical capabilities has had a profound impact on how and where health care is provided. Diagnosis and treatment have shifted from the traditional inpatient hospital setting to the outpatient setting. This move to the outpatient setting is not just an initiative of providers. Some see it as a response to a changing society that wants quick and convenient options.

Urgent care clinics have replaced hospital emergency rooms or waiting weeks until the next available opening with a busy primary care physician. Hospital administrators have witnessed a gradual shift of patient care to the fast-growing outpatient sector. It has been estimated that 60 percent of a hospital's revenue comes from inpatient care. Health care economists are projecting that, in the 1990s, this amount will decrease to about 30 percent. This projection has hospital administrators and boards rethinking their long-range strategic planning toward diversifying their health care delivery programs and becoming more outpatient oriented. This shift has also created a struggle for the control of outpatient care and ambulatory ancillary and therapeutic services between hospitals and doctors.

Physicians and hospitals both have ventured into the expanding outpatient market. Radiology (both diagnostic and therapeutic), clinical laboratory, hemodialysis, home infusion therapy, and ambulatory surgical procedures are but a few of the services hospitals and medical groups are competing to provide. Surgeons who, for example, cannot get enough operating room time at an affiliated hospital can now use local freestanding same-day surgery centers to keep up with growing patient demand. Hospitals used to be the only entities that could afford large and expensive radiology equipment. Advances in the technology, however, have created new imaging (magnetic resonance imaging and computerized tomography scanning) that receives high reimbursement, which makes it affordable for physicians to provide in their more convenient setting. Infusion therapy for nutrition, chemotherapy, or antibiotics can now follow the patient home from the hospital with hospital or medical group staff providing patient training and care in the patient's home.

In sum, hospital administrators must plan to compensate for the losses of inpatient business by either competing with physicians or joining with them.

Patients: The New Consumers of Health Care

The public is now finding itself in the middle of the struggle between hospitals, physicians, employers, and the major payers for the control of the health care market. Hospitals and physicians who realize that their patients are demanding choice, convenience, quality, and economy no longer take the public for granted, particularly if they must make major contributions to the cost of their care.

Employers have asked employees to contribute to the increased costs through more and greater copayments and deductible features. However, as health plan enrollees have contributed more, they have also demanded more for the money they spend. Physicians are beginning to encounter patients who are unwilling to wait more than 30 minutes in waiting rooms or who refuse to pay for failed procedures or services. Consumers are demanding that services be good or they will take their business elsewhere.

This consumerism has resulted in other unexpected outcomes. Theorists thought that managed care's restriction of patient freedom would lower utilization; however, patients have not been happy about their loss of freedom of choice. As a result, employees have begun to pressure employers to offer PPOs and other more traditional plan options that afford them freedom.

Physicians and hospitals are going to have to deal with this new consumerism. The public wants more accommodating health care delivery, whether it be at a hospital, in a physician's office, or at home. As a result, hospital and physician loyalty is being exchanged for convenience and lower out-of-pocket costs.

Conclusion

This chapter has discussed the market forces that are adversely influencing the control that hospitals and physicians have traditionally maintained over health care delivery. These forces are also creating competition between hospitals and physicians that, if not effectively managed, will drive them apart rather than together. Hospitals and physicians must find new responses to a consumer-oriented public that will attract and keep patient loyalty and market share. Service delivery must be looked at for quality, convenience, and comfort. Hospital administrators and physicians must decide who is in a better position to offer and deliver a particular service. They must realize that each must share the market for both to win.

4

VERTICAL INTEGRATION: THE SEARCH FOR NEW COMPETITIVE HEALTH CARE DELIVERY STRUCTURES

Chapters 2 and 3 described health care industry trends that have pressured hospitals and physicians to find new ways to deliver cost-effective health care. Hospitals have perhaps been more successful than physicians in responding to the financial realities of the trends. Hospital administrators have gradually expanded the mission of their hospitals beyond that of merely being a hospital to that of forming a core of a large network of providers that systematically capture business for their hospitals. In contrast physicians, for many reasons, have been less responsive to developing a new mission and are beginning to see their positions as esteemed controllers of health care delivery, their financial positions, and their autonomy eroded. This chapter discusses a major new countervailing response to the trends—that of joining hospitals with physicians to create a vertically integrated organization that promises to better position them for marketplace survival.

A New Approach to Marketplace Realities

Hospitals are developing a new approach to the marketplace. Hospital administrators and physicians are beginning to share a common philosophy and mission that take advantage of each other's strengths. The search for strategic advantage in the marketplace has led hospitals to incorporate physicians into the development and administration of jointly controlled health care delivery networks. Networking combined with traditional marketing of programs (see Figure 4.1) creates an expanded service area where the public receives the many types and levels of service that are needed right in its own backyard.

Networking acknowledges that hospitals and physicians serve the same clientele in the same territory and that the resulting territory often overlaps with those of their competitors. The result of networking is a much larger and more powerful marketing entity that reduces competition from other hospitals or physician-hospital organizations, thereby creating a more secure future. In sum, hospital administrators are developing vertically integrated organizations that include the direct participation of physicians in the systematic expansion of hospital interests beyond their immediate campus and market area (see Exhibit 4.1).

The development of vertically integrated networks begins with getting hospitals organized to be effective at pursuing the approach.

Figure 4.1   Vertically Integrated Hospital Organization Structure

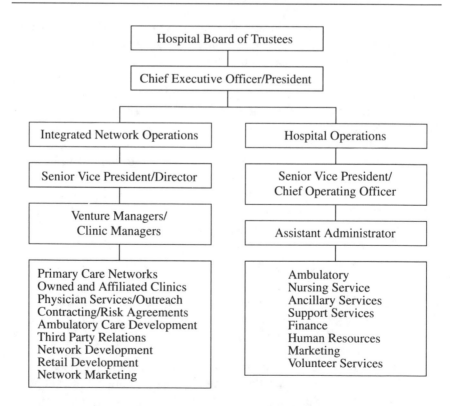

Exhibit 4.1 Possible Hospital/Physician Network Services

Pain management clinic	Back pain clinic
Wound healing	Women's health center
Gerontology program	Heart clinic
Diabetes center	Sports medicine clinic
Outpatient same-day surgery center	Kidney dialysis center
Intravenous therapy services	Cancer treatment
Hand therapy services	Allergy clinic
Weight loss program	Infertility clinic
MRI center	Therapeutic radiology
Arthritis clinic	Physical medicine
Childbirth and parenting programs	Lithotripsy center
Spinal cord injury center	Glaucoma screening

Expanding Hospital Organization Structure

Hospitals must develop organizational structures that support the networking of major new ventures with physicians. Hospitals and physicians have traditionally operated independently and in a rather symbiotic manner. Physicians have usually maintained their own offices and independence, expressed little interest in hospital operations, set up competing enterprises, and therefore been viewed as outsiders when seeing patients at hospitals. Similarly many hospital administrators, although recognizing that their medical staff is an integral part of their hospital, have run their hospital as though they are in business by themselves. Add to this situation untested beliefs that hospital administrators feel that they know how to run medical group practices and that physicians do not, and the stage is set for inherent and often undiscussable conflict.

It is easy to see why these conflicting positions and attitudes make it difficult for hospitals to make headway in joining with physicians to develop an integrated approach to marketplace survival. Nonetheless, many hospital administrators have begun to change their attitudes towards physicians and are campaigning for physician participation in building large, vertically integrated health care delivery networks that provide all levels of care. The cornerstone of hospital strategic planning now includes bonding the hospital with its medical staff to present the public with the image of a true partnership that serves the community. As will be discussed in Chapter 7, hospital administrators have developed a growing interest in medical group acquisitions, mergers, start-ups, and contract management services.

In sum, hospital governance and planning is beginning to exceed the traditional boundaries of a hospital's campus and immediate service area and is growing to include the total health care delivery service area where staff physicians practice medicine. This eventuality is requiring hospitals not only to develop an expanded notion of partnership with physicians but also to innovate new ways of structuring their administration.

Changing Traditional Hierarchy

Hospital administrative hierarchy has traditionally been designed to manage the operations of hospitals with little attention to meaningful physician involvement. Chief of staff and medical director positions have usually been limited to overseeing credentialing, medical staff, and patient care issues through committees. This approach, which limits physician involvement to managing their activities within the hospital, is now evolving to include physician participation in planning and managing internal and external aspects of the hospital's business.

Hospital administrators are adding new levels of administration that facilitate direct medical staff involvement. Director, assistant administrator, and even vice-president are positions that are being created for new departments such as physician services, medical staff relations, clinic management services, and medical outreach (Figure 4.2). These new positions and departments operationalize the interest of hospital administrators in developing direct physician participation in strategy and policy development and the managing of hospital operations. Their importance is often underscored by their direct reporting to the chief executive officer.

The decision to appoint a physician or an administrator to the position of vice-president or director is a critical one. Hospitals that are developing a network of physicians and services will need a person who has experience in managing health care delivery systems, including the development and operation of medical practices. The position will require hands-on expertise in managing medical office operations, physician-operated services such as physical therapy, and physician-owned enterprises like ambulatory surgery and imaging centers. Additionally, experience in resolving practice management issues and hospital–medical group liaison will be important. These skills will be particularly important when a financially distressed but important admitting medical group approaches the hospital for assistance. Experienced clinic and medical group managers or practice consultants who also have hospital-related experience can be likely candidates for the role. Networking also requires the involvement of a physician-administrator who can work behind the scenes to gain physician support and reduce the anxiety many physicians have in working with hospital administrators. It should be added that vertically integrated hospital–medical group networks lead to

Figure 4.2 Typical Hospital Organizational Structure for Physician Services Program

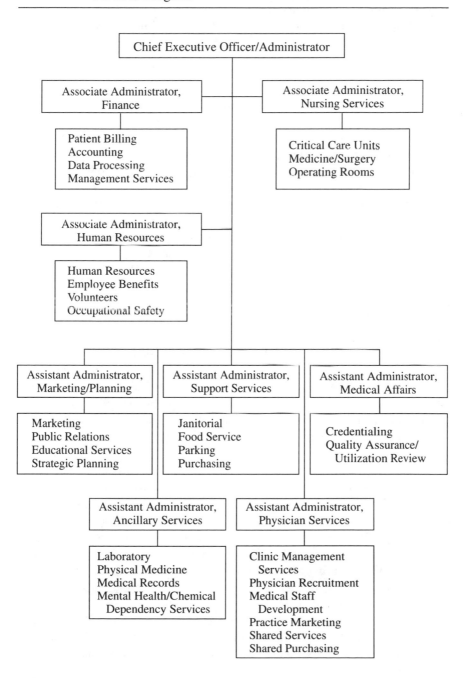

the creation of corporate entities to oversee these external activities, leaving hospital management to run their hospital. (The legal implications of separate corporate entities are discussed in Chapter 6.)

Hospitals that implement a network strategy must develop the right mix of primary and specialty care physicians to serve the needs of those in their expanded service area.

Networking Primary Care Physicians

Chapter 3 describes the growing importance of primary care physicians to managed care organizations. These physicians are the gatekeepers who control the flow of patients to hospitals and their specialist colleagues. Two or three large primary care groups (10–15 physicians) can serve 20,000 to 50,000 managed care enrollees in addition to tens of thousands of additional patients.

Hospital administrators who wish to network their way to an expanded geographic market area will find it easier to deal with a relatively small cadre of geographically dispersed primary care groups. Primary care medical groups must be located in the right place, serve the right patient and payer mix, and be able to be allied with the right HMOs and PPOs.

Networking primary care groups can take a number of forms. Hospitals can be asked to provide management assistance to improve operations and financial support to aid in growth related problems, such as developing new buildings and practice sites, physician recruitment, or the purchasing of new equipment. Hospitals can also provide financial stability to groups going through difficult times as a result of start-up problems, physician unrest and turnover, and declining payer mix. And last, hospitals can cooperate with primary care groups in absorbing some of the risks associated with managed care contracting.

Health maintenance organizations usually offer capitated risk-sharing arrangements to primary care groups. Groups that do not wish to assume all the financial risk can share it with a hospital that agrees to a set reimbursement schedule at a percentage of the capitation budgeted for hospital care. The sharing of risk assures physicians that they will not be at complete risk for financial problems related to unexpected utilization arising from adverse patient selection. Sharing risk with primary care groups is in the best interest of a hospital that might otherwise lose the enrollees if they are reassigned to a medical group affiliated with another hospital.

In sum, if a hospital wants to stay competitive in the 1990s, it must be attentive to the needs of its affiliated primary care groups. They must be kept thriving and happily bonded to ensure a steady flow of admissions.

Networking Specialty Physicians

The value of family physicians and general practitioners to managed care has not deterred hospital administrators from also devoting attention to specialty physicians who have patients who often consume large volumes of hospital services. Hospital administrators realize that, if they are to have thriving inpatient and specialty services, they need specialists who are in high demand among hospitals. The reason for the competition lies in the fact that specialists can more easily transfer their loyalties to different hospitals than primary care physicians who have patients who may choose to change physicians to stay with a certain program or hospital. In contrast, patients of specialists often develop considerable dependence on their expertise, such as might be the case with a diabetic patient, and will follow their doctors to new locations. In sum, specialists are more flexible in choosing a hospital or outpatient facility with which to work. As a result, hospitals have to make sure that these physicians have the resources that they need to keep productive, which usually translates into keeping up with the latest technology. Surgeons, cardiologists, and obstetricians must be satisfied with the operating rooms, intensive care units, and radiology and laboratory services to maintain their loyalty to a hospital.

Additionally, greater competition for patients who have special needs is forcing medical groups to establish multiple practice sites to capture the patient volume they need to fulfill their income and practice expectations. The development of multiple sites often causes medical groups to cross over into the territories of other hospitals, which fuels competition between hospitals for the medical group's business. The hospital that best caters to the physicians will tend to win most of their business. Facilities such as operating rooms (ORs) and OR time for surgeons, birthing programs and units for obstetricians, high-technology coronary care units for cardiologists, and a hospital staff that is responsive to physician needs are all examples of what these physicians expect and what hospitals must deliver.

Specialty physicians are also important to hospitals that wish to expand their service areas. Specialists are usually welcome guests in underserved areas, and specialists can often work with local primary care groups to provide sites for their practices. This type of relationship creates a win-win situation. People in the underserved area are better served and do not have a long drive to a specialist's office. The specialty physicians secure more business to meet income expectations, and they also gain the respect and appreciation of those served. The primary care physicians improve their image in the community and spread some of their overhead costs to a larger practice base that now includes specialty care. The networked hospital gains more admissions and better utilization of its high-technology diagnostic and therapeutic equipment and develops a marketing presence in the new service area. Last, local hospitals usually also benefit from referrals for services that they have available, services that are consumed in a larger volume by the patients of specialists.

The win-win outcome also occurs when the specialists are networked with a large tertiary care hospital. Local primary care physicians appreciate the availability of specialists and their center's technology. They feel assured that their patients are seeing a top-flight specialist and will have immediate access to a state-of-the-art tertiary care facility. And, should a trip to the tertiary care hospital be necessary, their patient will be followed by his or her own specialist whom he or she knows and trusts.

It is also important to appreciate that many areas of the country might only have a university hospital that serves as a regional tertiary care center. Equally important to appreciate is that most of the physicians in the area might be graduates of the university's medical school and will want to maintain close ties to the faculty and the school's continuing education programs. Networking with these physicians must not threaten these important linkages. And last, large multispecialty groups that offer both primary care and specialty care usually need to affiliate with university and teaching hospitals to handle complex tertiary care services such as cardiovascular surgery, organ transplantation, oncology treatment, burn care, and treatment for spinal cord injuries.

The issues for specialty tertiary care in large, urban, university teaching hospitals is somewhat different. They are finding they must strengthen their relationships with primary care physicians or face the possibility of developing their own cadre of primary care physicians and clinics that compete with their own admitting physicians. Maintaining market share creates a hard-to-resolve dilemma. Unlike their private practice counterparts, who accept the inevitability of head-on competition, large, often state-funded, medical school practices need to protect their "town/gown" balance. Networking can be an effective low-profile approach to joining with local area physicians without engendering distrust and feelings of unfair competition.

Developing New Hospital-Physician Networking Structures

The major advantage of developing networks is their ability to negotiate with employers who are turning to self-insurance. Networks provide health care delivery at competitive costs by cutting out the intermediary, the managed care plans. They permit package pricing that includes physician and hospital fees in one price, which puts pressure on the networked hospital and physicians to manage costs.

There are two general approaches to developing new hospital-physician networking structures. The first involves the actual envelopment of medical group practices by a hospital. In this scenario, the practice becomes fully integrated into the hospital's management structure. The relationship is one that involves the direct involvement of hospital administrators in the operation of a group practice as a result of purchasing the practice, jointly owning it, or providing contracted management services for its operation.

The second approach involves developing new legal entities—physician-hospital organizations (PHOs) or independent practice associations (IPAs). Physician-hospital organizations are relatively new. They give hospital administrators and physicians a formal role in the development of a joint organization governed by a board of directors, preferably involving equal representation of hospital administration and the physicians. Independent practice associations were initially designed to jointly pursue marketing their services to health plans and other major health care purchasers while maintaining control over their practices and independence from hospitals. Independent practice associations have more recently grown to include hospitals sharing their resources and working jointly on mutual interests at arm's length.

Both approaches permit physicians to network with a hospital and other medical groups to better compete in the marketplace. They also provide a balanced organizational structure where neither the hospital nor the physician groups dominate. As a result adversarial relationships between primary care and specialty physicians, particularly in relation to reimbursement and the utilization of services, are avoided. And last, both approaches provide a basis for developing effective leadership, good communications, and strategies that serve all members.

A last consideration worthy of mention is the relationship between structure and reimbursement. The structure of the venture determines who can bill and collect for services. Joint ventures where a separate legal entity is not created require each party to bill separately. However, this approach might not always maximize combined reimbursement. In some instances it might be better to structure the network as a separate legal entity, have the hospital employ the physicians, and bill for all services or, conversely, to have the physicians bill for all services rendered. Naturally, safe harbor legislation must be carefully checked for potential violations as innovative network agreements are developed (see Chapter 6). In sum, reimbursement methodology should be carefully considered when forming any type of joint relationship.

Marketing Hospital-Physician Services: Centers of Excellence

Competition has forced hospitals and physicians to find ways to distinguish themselves from their competitors. Hospitals are responding by networking with medical groups to create centers of excellence. The networked hospital and physicians create a new marketing entity, one that is structured to provide specialized, comprehensive, cost-effective, and convenient services for patients. A hospital and physician–sponsored diabetes center might, for example, include a broad spectrum of services such as patient education, family support, and access to state-of-the-art clinical research and experimental drug therapies (see Exhibit 4.1).

Another good example of this approach is a cancer center. In this case, oncologists and the hospital combine to provide expertise, ancillary services (radiology, pathology, nuclear medicine, physical therapy), space, and support staff to form an integrated product line that provides patients with one-stop shopping. Additionally, hospital support staff provide patient education, counseling services, home health care, and hospice services to further meet patient needs. This planned integration of services creates a compelling reason why patients will wish to use the center while the center approach also provides a pleasing setting for physicians and staff to work in.

Hospital administrators must, when setting up one of these ventures, be careful to not alienate physicians who are not involved with the venture. These centers can achieve a high level of community recognition, which can threaten medical staff who have been excluded. To be avoided is developing a center that, at the outset, appears to involve only a select group of physicians. Care must be taken to avoid the development of hostile attitudes that can spill over to affect relations between the hospital and the remainder of its medical staff.

It is also important to appreciate that physician motivations for joining with a hospital in developing a center might differ somewhat from those of the hospital's administration. The physicians will see the development of the center as an important contributor to their incomes, whereas the hospital might see it as an opportunity to better utilize its ancillary services and beds—a difference that might cause the hospital not to pursue the profit-making aspect of the joint venture with as much gusto as the physicians. This break-even mentality on the part of hospital administrators can also create unfair competition for other physician-owned enterprises, which can serve to unnecessarily alienate them.

Network Strategic Planning

Hospital and physician groups that are going to work together to develop new health care delivery ventures must be prepared to plan, something hospitals are often staffed to support. Like in obtaining a certificate of need, the two parties need to determine whether the market will support the proposed venture. Hospitals should determine both the demand for the product line as well as the interest of physician groups in the new service venture. They must keep in mind the growing evidence that the competitive environment for ventures in outpatient surgery centers, lithotripsy, and MRI is straining relationships between the hospitals and their medical staff members, who often form their own partnerships to provide these services.

Conclusion

Hospital administrators who want to secure and expand their service area are now trying to accomplish this expansion by creating networks with physicians that permit the development of large, high-technology, comprehensive, highly visible programs and centers. Networking is proving to be an effective method of marketing and countervails the purchasing power of managed care plans and employers.

5

Integrated Strategic Planning for Hospitals and Medical Groups

The last three chapters have reminded hospital administrators that patients are becoming more informed about their health and the health care delivery system. Patients expect more and demand more. Competition for patients has increased between hospitals, between physicians, and between freestanding labs and services. Add to this competition constantly shifting political, legal, and reimbursement policies, and the necessity for strategic planning becomes apparent. There is just too much complexity and too much at stake to not know what a hospital or medical group is trying to accomplish. Joint hospital and medical group strategic planning is essential in gaining the synergy that should result in linking medical groups to hospitals. This chapter examines what it takes for a hospital to contribute to the strategic planning for medical group practices and how to coordinate the planning with the hospital's plans.

Strategic planning has come to mean marketing. Linking hospital marketing practices with those of physician practices is the focus of this chapter. Maintaining and expanding market share is the new reality for physicians, who previously did not view themselves as subject to the rigors of the marketplace.

Medical Staff Development: The Cornerstone for Hospital Strategic Planning in the 1990s

If managed care and provider payment reform were the health care revolution of the 1980s, then the development of expanded service delivery areas and direct involvement of medical staff in hospital operations might well become the focus for health care providers in the 1990s. Hospitals that wish to take the lead in the marketplace will have to develop a large, comprehensive, complex, vertically integrated, networked health care delivery system that must include physician participation to work. Primary care physicians will become the foundation for developing networked, geographically dispersed primary care clinics to serve a vastly expanded catchment area. Specialty physicians will also fill the important role of ensuring that the specialty needs of the service area are met.

Doing nothing is not an option. Hospital administrators must make sure that their affiliated medical groups are vital and growing.

Many hospital administrators who are aggressively pursuing medical staff development might not hesitate to circumvent an existing physician or medical group that balks at working with them. In this case, the hospital is forced into a position of fostering competition within its medical staff at the risk of succumbing to the political pressure of a particular physician or medical group. However, an additional risk is another hospital moving in to supply the needed services, thus hurting all the parties who might have been linked to that resistant physician or medical group.

However, success does hinge on not alienating staff physicians by continually acting unilaterally. The key to success lies in the hospital's ability to show its physicians that their markets are basically the same and that a networked health care system approach will work to everyone's advantage.

The remainder of this chapter discusses medical group strategic planning and linkages to hospital-based resources and planning.

Market Oriented Analysis for Medical Groups

Strategic planning for medical groups involves a number of steps not unlike those relied on by the planning staffs of hospitals. Medical group strategic planning starts with a market-oriented analysis that consists of three steps: the market audit, strategy formulation, and the selection of a marketing mix and tactics. Each step operationalizes the one before. It is important to realize physicians might not appreciate that a plan that cannot be implemented is no plan at all.

The Market Audit

A market audit is a systematic review of the operating environment of a medical group and the group's attributes in terms of its ability to provide services and an appraisal of the group's current marketing activities. The audit should clarify the medical group's mission statement, goals, and objectives and examine them for their internal consistency and how they relate to existing plans and hospital plans.

A hospital's marketing staff can facilitate the audit. It is advantageous, when evaluating whether to develop a linking relationship with a medical group, to have a clear idea of what the group's mission, goals, and objectives are and where they are compatible with those of the hospital's, where they conflict, and whether the conflicts can be reconciled. This understanding is also a critical first step in developing the desired synergy.

A market audit involves a comprehensive analysis of both external market conditions and internal factors related to marketing. Exhibits 5.1 and 5.2 provide examples of the questions that need to be answered. Exhibit 5.1 lists pertinent questions about a medical group's external operating environment. Exhibit 5.2 is designed to assess a medical group's internal operating environment. One might readily observe from the two tables that most medical groups can benefit from help that a hospital's trained staff can provide. It is also likely the hospital's planners already possess much of the information about the community and region, and the medical group does not need to independently duplicate it.

Strategy Formulation for Medical Groups

Strategy formulation for medical groups involves finding a market position that takes advantage of the group's attributes while also defending against competitors. Strategy formulation is the delineation of the medical group's mission, goals, and objectives and a description of how the group will operate to fulfill them.

In the new highly competitive environment, medical group strategy formulation should include both offensive and defensive actions that exploit marketplace opportunities and deal with competitors. Three traditional approaches to market positioning apply to medical practices—collaboration, diversification, and servicing an ecological niche.

Before discussing these approaches it should be noted that a hospital's planning staff can help to assess the approaches to market positioning being considered. It must be clear how the medical group will implement its mission, goals, and objectives and whether the strategies selected are feasible. A hospital's staff should have the expertise to handle the assessment while maintaining important objectivity. Additionally, the review also enables planners to find cross-compatibilities with the hospital's strategies that, if joined with those of the medical group, will improve a strategy or permit new strategies to be considered.

Hospital-Physician Collaboration

Exhibit 5.1   External Marketing Assessment

Assessment of the macro-operating environment

What are the trends in the following areas and their anticipated impact on medical group operations?

- Changing demographics
- Changing consumer values
- Changing reimbursement methods
- Changing economic conditions
- Changing labor market

- Changing access to capital
- Changing technology
- Changing political climate
- Changing government regulation
- Changing legal climate

Assessment of the immediate marketplace

What are the medical group's characteristics in the following areas?
- Geographic market
- Patient mix by age and payer
- Relationship to its patients (loyalty)
- Relationship with major employers
- Relationship with referring physicians (age, type of practice)
- Relationship to managed care programs

Is it possible to consider segmenting the medical group's market either geographically by county, city, or zip code or demographically by age, sex, family size, income, occupation, insurer, or diagnostic codes?

What are the unserved needs to the medical group's service area by market segment?

What governs consumer decision making in the choice of physician?

Assessment of local competition

Who are the major competitors?
How large or powerful are they?
What is their service area?
What types of services are offered?
What is their referral pattern?
How successful are they?
Are they growing in size and in the services they offer?
What are their existing relationships with each other and area hospitals?
What appears to be each competitor's marketing strategy?
What are each competitor's strengths and weaknesses?
Is it likely new competitors will enter the market?

Source: Adapted with permission of Business Word Inc. from K.D. Bopp and S. Allcorn, "Medical Group Management: A Marketing Orientation," in the September 1986 issue of *Health Care Strategic Management*, Englewood, CO. Copyright 1986, all rights reserved.

Exhibit 5.2   Internal Marketing Assessment

Assessment of medical group mission, organization, and management

What is the stated mission of the medical group?
- What services does it claim to offer?
- What does it claim is its market area and interest to consumers?
- What goals are set for the staff in providing services?
- Are they consistent with the mission?
- Have goals been broken down into a list of objectives?
- Who is responsible for monitoring progress toward fulfilling the goals?

How is the medical group organized?
- Is there a formal organization chart?
- Are there written bylaws for governance?
- Who are the key figures in decision making?
- Are decision makers adequately empowered?
- How many sites are there?

How well managed is the medical group?
- What types of plans have been developed and how well documented are they?
- Are there any chronic operating or interpersonal problems in the group?
- Who has final authority for daily decision making?
- What types of information systems are in use and how adequate are they?
- How well conceived are the service delivery systems?
- Are there formal position descriptions where appropriate?

Assessment of human resources management

How many staff are there?
Are they adequately oriented and trained?
What are the ages and skills of the physicians?
What efforts are made toward staff development?
What types of benefits does the group offer?
What are the attitudes of the group's members toward the following features of the practice:
- Their operating environment
- The mission and goals of the group
- Performance measures
- Each other and patients
- Management
- Their salaries and benefits

Continued

Exhibit 5.2 Continued

Assessment of facilities and equipment

> How do the group's facilities and equipment compare to that of other medical groups?
> Is the equipment in good repair?
> What technology is being used or is anticipated to be used?
> Is the location of the group's practice adequate?
> Is the size of the facility appropriate?
> Are facility costs reasonable?

Assessment of medical group financial management

> • How profitable is the group?
> • Does the group own assets other than accounts receivable?
> • Does the group have a debt structure?
> • Does the group have adequate internal control over its assets?
> • How are its books kept?

Source: Adapted with permission of Business Word Inc. from K.D. Bopp and S. Allcorn, "Medical Group Management: A Marketing Orientation," in the September 1986 issue of *Health Care Strategic Management*, Englewood, CO. Copyright 1986, all rights reserved.

Collaboration

The first market positioning approach involves negotiating collaborative arrangements with competitors and in particular with the networking hospital. Successful collaboration increases a medical group's power in the marketplace by resolving uncertainty in its favor. Collaboration takes four forms. Before continuing, it is important to mention a medical group should keep its legal counsel informed of its actions to be certain to avoid entering into any illegal or legally gray areas where competition is threatened. The legal implications of cooperation and the other types of collaboration that follow are also discussed elsewhere in this book. The discussion in this chapter serves to position concepts such as joint ventures relative to strategic planning.

Cooperation. Cooperation is defined as an effort to develop relationships with other providers for the purpose of jointly accomplishing the goals of the providers. This type of informal working relationship gives the advantage to the best managed medical group. For example, two medical groups or a group and a hospital might agree to share a parking lot or office space on alternate days to support the development of specialized clinics of interest to each participant.

Cooperation is an excellent place for a hospital to start building a linkage with a medical group. The relationship is voluntary and limited and can be easily terminated, something both partners might be interested in at the beginning. However, the scope of the projects undertaken should not be unnecessarily restricted. The working relationship should be jointly monitored for problems and for creeping change toward one of the following strategies since a successful relationship will evolve toward taking advantage of more opportunities.

Coordination. Coordination involves two or more providers agreeing to adjust their actions relative to each other to attain a collective goal. Several providers might, for example, work together to develop an advertising campaign to promote the benefits of regular physical examinations. The participating providers benefit from the effort, which might not have been undertaken by one medical group acting alone.

Coordination is a more planned and binding step for hospitals and medical groups to take and may be perceived as threatening by some physicians. On the other hand, there are many advantages to developing a formal working relationship to pursue a specified marketing strategy, and these should be emphasized. Care should be exercised in laying out who is responsible for what, what kind of funding and other resources will be expected on the part of each provider, and the distribution of any incremental income that can be construed to be jointly earned. The terms of the agreement should specify a clear scope that delimits the enterprise, the time period involved, and how the enterprise will be evaluated.

Cooptation. Cooptation involves absorbing new operating elements into a current structure to stay competitive. A medical group might add a new service or change a policy as a direct response to changes competitors have made. Taking on the attributes of other medical groups that have successfully innovated change makes the coopting group more competitive.

Hospital planners and administrators should be alert for opportunities to modify the hospital's operations based on what is learned from working with medical groups. However, hospital administrators must be aware that the physicians might become suspicious and fearful. A hospital that picks up something from a medical group should discuss it with the physicians before using it. Similarly, the physicians might view the advocacy of a potentially useful hospital operating element for a medical group with skepticism. It might not work in a different and smaller setting or fit the values system the medical group has developed. Cooptation also opens up the possibility for a hospital-linked medical group to take on an operating element of a local competitor that could not have been considered without the support of the hospital. For example, a medical group might develop a preferred provider contract with the help and guidance of the staff of the hospital.

Merger. Merger involves two or more providers coming under common control (of one or the other or a third party). Merger improves market power, as is illustrated by the need for antitrust laws. The merger of a hospital with a medical group and its facilities and auxiliary enterprises can be considered as an effective strategy for competing in the marketplace. Hospitals might wish to buy out existing practices, develop formal long-term management contracts with them, or perhaps even start their own practice groups to achieve the advantages this level of collaboration offers. The acquisition of medical groups will be discussed more fully in Chapter 11.

Diversification

Diversification is a marketing strategy that reduces a practice's dependence on one market. Practices can enter new marketing domains to improve their likelihood of success. A marketing domain consists of claims a medical group makes in terms of the products or services it offers or the population it serves. Diversification involves expansion into related market domains or completely different ones. A medical group might open a satellite clinic, pharmacy, nursing home, or physical therapy center or offer home care or possibly purchase a car dealership. Diversification can also involve vertical integration where the medical group moves into another domain of health care delivery. For example, a medical group might form its own PPO to secure a presence in the managed health care marketplace and reduce dependence on HMO participation.

Diversification offers hospital administrators many opportunities to develop synergistic linkages with medical groups. For example, hospitals often expand into developing practice buildings for physicians. Other examples are the development of new testing and therapeutic services to support specialized practices or the development of a clinic at an alternate site in conjunction with a practice in the area. These kinds of opportunities are only limited by imagination. Other common examples are the development of smoking cessation programs, physician-supervised diet programs, wellness programs, executive physical programs, nursing home facilities, and specialized living facilities for the elderly and the operation of therapy and fitness centers.

Hospitals and practices will find many opportunities to collaborate on diversification projects as each brings important resources to the bargaining table. Joint efforts to diversify into, for example, diagnostic centers, home health care, or nursing homes reduces and spreads the risks while facilitating the timely development of plans that can be readily implemented. As a result, everyone, including the surrounding community, stands to benefit from diversification that provides better and more health care resources.

Ecological Niche

An ecological niche is defined in strict marketing terms as the capacity of a practice to carve out a niche in the marketplace where competitors either cannot follow (because of entry barriers) or will not follow (because of a response barrier). Typical entry barriers are high costs of entry, a lack of access to unique or scarce resources, and geographic distance. Response barriers typically include the likely response of practices already occupying the niche, which might include additional advertising, the expansion of services, and price cutting. As long as competitors stay out of the niche, it can be exploited to the practice's advantage. There are three categories of ecological niches that apply equally well to linking arrangements between hospitals and practices.

Overall cost leadership. Achieving a low-cost position (for example a PPO contract) can make it unprofitable for competitors to respond. For a practice to achieve a low-cost position, considerable attention needs to be directed to increasing operating efficiency to reduce the costs, to avoiding costs of marginal consumers, and to minimizing unnecessary expenses such as travel to unnecessary meetings.

Linkage with a hospital can lower costs, as discussed in Chapters 4 and 9. Linkage may also create economies of scale that permit one-stop shopping and packaged services that provide lower overall time and costs to consumers and third parties. A consideration already mentioned is the possibility of combining resources to make competitive bids for PPOs or possibly forming an HMO, both of which are low-cost positions. Hospital administrators can also contribute to a practice's cost effectiveness by analyzing operating costs and systems, reviewing staffing, and exploring compatible cost-minimizing connections with the hospital, which might, for example, include low-cost accounting, purchasing, and billing services.

Differentiation. Differentiation involves being seen to be different from other practices. Typical areas of differentiation for practices are image, reputation, technology used in practice, unique specialized services, and quality of service. Successful differentiation insulates a medical group from other groups by developing consumer loyalty that reduces consumer sensitivity to the actions of competitors.

Hospitals can facilitate medical group differentiation by, for example, providing public acknowledgement of an association with the hospital, the development of a jointly sponsored clinic near the hospital, or the development of a joint communitywide program, all of which can make the medical group appear bigger than life and striving for excellence in community service.

Hospitals are in an excellent position to provide medical group patients convenient access to sophisticated hospital services, which has the effect of bringing the medical group under the marketing and image management efforts of the hospital. Medical groups that have priority access for their patients will have a service and marketing edge that provides their patients the appearance of one-stop shopping in a state-of-the-art health care mall-like environment.

Focus. Focus is based on the notion that a medical group can serve a narrow market segment better than a broad segment or a number of segments. This approach involves serving a particular buyer group (such as children, women, or the aged), a service need (such as cardiac catheterization or eating disorders), or a particular geographic area. This strategy assumes that through focus, differentiation and cost leadership can be accomplished.

Hospitals can help linking medical groups to become more focused by developing complementary resources and programs that permit a group to function effectively within a narrow band of service. For example, a hospital might seek to develop regional leadership in cardiac medicine, geriatrics, or the care of premature infants and locate a medical group that is willing to work with the hospital in developing the service. At the same time, many medical groups arc highly focused in such areas as sports medicine, pediatrics, or gynecology and can provide the hospital important opportunities to focus on service areas that might have been neglected. Neither the hospital nor the medical group could do it without the other, and the medical group involved gains the added benefit of avoiding the risk of placing all its eggs into one basket by the hospital's willingness to support the medical group's efforts and to help it refocus at a later date if necessary.

The selection of one or more marketing strategies leads to the problem of how to implement them.

Marketing Mix and Tactics

Medical groups must figure out how to best implement the marketing strategies selected. Operating variables such as service design (convenience clinics, for example), clinic locations, pricing, types and number of services offered, and promotional activities must be examined for their contribution to a successful implementation. Additional organizational development that facilitates the accomplishment of the mission, goals, and objectives by improving the medical group's capacity to execute its strategy must also be anticipated.

There are many marketing mix and tactical decisions that a hospital's staff can aid a medical group in developing and that can also be coordinated with those of the hospital to gain competitive advantage. Every avenue of pursuit should be explored.

Service Designs

Service design involves determining the core consumer benefit. For the patient the core benefits are hope, relief from pain and suffering, and good service delivered in a pleasant manner and atmosphere. To ensure these core benefits are delivered, a service blueprint should be developed to manage the services that provide the benefits. Service blueprinting includes (1) creating a flowchart of all the steps in rendering patient care services with particular attention given to the not-so-obvious aspects of the services; (2) identifying potential problems with processes, personnel, and systems; and (3) determining the time involved with each service while (4) also relating the effectiveness with which services provide the core benefits to the overall operating efficiency and profitability of the medical group. Patients should be observed as they pass through the waiting room to clinic rooms, to laboratories and back to clinic rooms. Also to be observed are how billing, collection, and departure are handled. Problems can be uncovered such as patients having to routinely give up their clothes on entering clinic rooms regardless of their complaint and then being expected to walk about in the clinic in unsightly, uncomfortable, revealing, and drafty gowns. This type of treatment humiliates patients, who will not be eager to return.

In sum, patients are attentive to how they are treated and to the appearance of the facilities. These are often the only aspects of their visit on which they base their judgment to return. Even though they might have received outstanding care, the lack of considerate service can cause them not to return. And worse yet, they will tell their friends about how they were treated and spread negative word of mouth. Hospital staff can provide the objectivity, expertise, and staff time to perform this much needed service design work, which can be wisely expanded to include the services that the hospital provides the medical group's patients.

Distribution

Distribution considerations involve how a medical group reaches its target market economically. There are two practice distribution channels. Direct distribution involves providing services where and when they are needed by the consumer. Direct distribution includes convenient hours of operation, satellite clinics, mobile clinics, nursing home coverage, and house calls. Indirect distribution involves relying on an intermediate step, which is, in the case of medical groups, referring physicians. A hospital's staff can be most helpful in perfecting and fine tuning these distribution channels for a medical group. For example, a hospital can contribute resources to the development of additional clinics and services or develop and market a convenient referring physician program for participating medical groups. During the 1980s hospitals also began to employ direct sales forces to sell services to mass consumers such as employers, insurance companies, and organizations involved with various forms of prepayment. These efforts can be expanded to include medical groups that, when networked with the hospital, provide the hospital more services to sell.

Price

During the 1970s, price was not a major element in the health care industry. Cost reimbursement was the norm. Price, however, became a major factor in the 1980s and will remain one of the most important factors in the future. Price is a function of cost and the profit motive. Already discussed is the use of price to establish low-price leadership. It was also noted that medical groups that cannot or do not want to compete based on low price can pursue other strategies such as focus and market differentiation that limit the price sensitivity of major buyers, third parties, and consumers. However, medical groups cannot ignore pricing considerations and remain competitive.

A hospital's staff has the experience and expertise to provide medical groups much needed information on pricing and reimbursement trends for medical services. A hospital's staff can also offer a medical group opportunities to develop more services to bill for, thereby spreading costs over a larger income base and permitting the medical group to bill at a lower overall level for its services. Hospital billing personnel might also be able to find ways to optimize charge capture, billing, and collection to further increase income from existing work.

Promotion

Promotion involves all efforts to communicate a positive image of a medical group to the public. Promotion includes advertising, publicity, personal contact, and direct sales efforts such as offering blood pressure screening clinics in shopping malls. All these elements of a marketing program are discussed below.

Advertising. Advertising decisions can be complex. They require the selection of the message and media and the making of decisions based on the demographic attributes of the target markets. Advertising can take many forms. Radio, television, newspaper, and yellow pages advertising are among the most common. Practices often advertise their location and services. Advertising is usually combined with other promotional efforts such as the offering of free clinics and educational opportunities. Advertising can also be directed toward referring physicians in the form of solicitous communications, announcements, and service promotions. Hospitals usually have staff that can aid medical groups in their use of advertising, but more important they can coordinate joint efforts to develop advertising campaigns with, if necessary, the assistance of consultants paid for by the hospital.

Publicity. Publicity can be effective but requires acquiring favorable coverage from uncontrollable media. However, newspapers and local radio and television stations can be managed into providing favorable coverage that might, for example, include regular coverage of free screening clinics and patient care success stories. However, care must also be taken to minimize negative coverage should a medical group encounter a problem such as a malpractice suit that reaches the public's attention. A hospital's public relations and marketing staff can combine forces with a medical group to develop newsworthy programs.

Public relations. Direct contact with consumers and referring physicians is yet another promotion opportunity. Public relations involves a broad range of activities such as contributions to community fund raising, the offering of free services or educational opportunities, participation in civic organizations and local clubs and practices, and the sponsoring of physical fitness programs or running or bicycling events. It is important to exploit every opportunity to present the medical group, its physicians, and its staff in a positive light to the public. Another public relations opportunity is providing the media a list of health care experts who can be interviewed as needs arise. Seasonal health care problems such as allergies, sunburn, and problems associated with cold weather can, for example, be brought to the attention of the media with information and interview opportunities provided. Announcements of changes in service or the addition of a new physician are also newsworthy. All these activities provide favorable publicity and interactions with the public that will hopefully cause members of the public to think of the medical group the next time a health care need arises. Public relations efforts can be enhanced by merging them, where appropriate, with those of a networking hospital. Costs can be shared and new opportunities developed that neither the hospital nor the medical group could achieve individually.

Direct sales. Direct sales efforts entail the creation of needs and wants in the minds of consumers that will cause them to seek their gratification. Motivation can be provided by developing special incentives for consumers to seek services such as free screening clinics, educational news releases, discounts, and one-time opportunities to receive a special package of services, a free service, or a service temporarily offered at a remote location. Combining the promotional resources of a medical group and a hospital can be especially effective if it is well managed. Hospitals can be especially effective at developing a long-term promotional strategy that takes advantage of what both a medical group and the hospital have to offer. Direct sales representatives or existing hospital staff can also be used to market the medical group to local employers and other large purchasers of health care services as part of a joint health care program. Programs such as executive physicals and industrial health care can provide medical groups and hospitals good income opportunities that can be added to a medical group's activities with little difficulty. These programs also serve to attract families to the sponsoring medical group and hospital for their health care. The development of practice-based contractual discounts to large users of health care services such as corporations is also an example where marketing in the form of direct sales can achieve the enrollment of employees.

Networked medical groups and hospitals must learn to manage these marketing mix concepts and tactics. Once a mix of services are selected for a medical group and the tactics are developed to market them, attention must be turned to ensuring that the medical group and its staff are able to offer the advertised high quality, consumer-oriented services. To do that they must develop an organization able to do a good job of providing the services being marketed.

Marketing Administration

Marketing involves all efforts by a medical group to achieve positive public recognition to promote the utilization of its services. This definition includes a number of already discussed promotional elements: advertising, publicity, public relations, and direct sales. It also includes the consideration of such things as keeping track of the costs of the marketing program's development and determining its cost effectiveness. Hospital administrators should encourage medical groups to keep complete and accurate records of plans and tactics to permit subsequent evaluation. The tactics should be clearly consistent with the goals and objectives of the medical group and include quantifiable objectives for measuring expected results. A medical group should not find that a particular service or aspect of the practice is being vigorously marketed when the group has not made it a goal to do so. It is also critical to develop a process for managing a formal marketing program. The following sections discuss some of the more important aspects of managing a medical group's marketing program.

Budgeting for Marketing

Depending on the marketing mix and tactics a medical group selects, considerable funding and other resources can be devoted to marketing. In particular, attention should be given to identifying all activities that are felt to be marketing oriented. A full and accurate accounting of these efforts is worthwhile to appreciate their cost, to spot ways of improving their effectiveness and efficiency, and to spot missed opportunities.

There are no guidelines or industry standards that inform a medical group how much to invest in marketing. However, expenditures should be informed by common sense assessments of costs and benefits. The budget can also be evaluated as a percent of total revenues, and, in this regard, available information on what to invest in marketing a medical group indicates that an appropriate level of expenditure is in the range of 5 to 10 percent of billings.

Linkage with a hospital will substantially reduce a medical group's marketing costs. Hospitals have completed marketing research that will generalize to a group and therefore need not be duplicated. Formal planning of marketing linkages can also lead to a hospital providing staff and other resources to aid a medical group in planning, all of which reduces the costs while improving the quality of the planning process.

The Marketing Committee

Large multispecialty practices should create a marketing committee to develop plans, monitor costs, and direct the marketing effort. The committee should be led by the director of strategic planning and composed of physicians and management staff who are interested in marketing and stakeholders from the departments to be marketed. Adequate support staff should be available for recording minutes, handling computers, and facilitating studies and analyses. Small medical groups routinely involve all physicians and administrators in planning and marketing activities, creating a marketing committee by default. Any medical group with a committee will benefit from the ad hoc membership of hospital administrators who are familiar with marketing.

Market Research

Good strategic planning involves considerable research. Market research needs to be carried out to determine trends in patient and community demographics and to determine market share by geographic area. There are many sources of market-related information. States, counties, and large cities collect information on the rates of admission; occupancy rates; the incidence of disease; and planned expansions of hospital services, plant, and equipment. National organizations such as the AMA, the Medical Group Management Association, and agencies of the federal government develop insightful analyses and reports. Information on the local market, if not derived from sources such as the above, requires specially designed studies. Here again the market research staff of a hospital can provide already developed information that helps to guide gathering additional information. Research must also be carried out on a medical group to understand its strengths and weaknesses and to gain a better appreciation of what is involved in positioning the group in the marketplace. Professional assistance to perform this research can be contracted for or provided by the hospital. Assistance is especially recommended to maintain objectivity. It is also particularly difficult to prepare integrated plans for medical groups that offer a variety of services. The help of an experienced hospital planner or a consultant can be particularly helpful in this regard.

Information and Decision Support

Care should be taken to preserve the content of strategic planning. Deliberations and information supporting decisions should be safeguarded to ensure the processes can be reconstructed should questions or problems arise. The collected data should be organized for preferably computerized storage and retrieval. Good records also assist those joining the effort (including consultants) to orient themselves.

Evaluation. Practices that invest substantial amounts in external marketing should seriously consider finding a means to evaluate the success of their marketing program. There are methods that can be used to uncover how effective an advertising campaign or other promotional effort has been. The return of coupons and telephone or mail surveys can yield insights into the return on investment of the marketing dollar. Evaluation depends on previously developed goals and measurable objectives against which progress can be compared. Provision must have been made for the collection and assembly of data and information on the results of the marketing efforts. Complete, accurate, timely, and representative information is critical in making evaluations. Evaluation should be considered when plans are originally made. For example, efforts to present public classes on skin cancer might be accompanied by the handing out of coupons for a discounted or free examination. These coupons can then be counted to determine the number of visits generated by the effort. A further step could be taken to correlate income generated for the medical group and the hospital by the patients that were acquired as a result of the classes. Evaluation implies corrective action when results do not meet objectives. Medical groups must be encouraged to constantly search for more effective ways of marketing while eliminating uneconomical and ineffective marketing strategies.

Contracting for marketing services. Contracts should be handled with care. It should be clear what services are being contracted for and at what cost, how contractual arrangements can be modified or terminated, and what outcomes will be produced in the specified times. Obtaining good services can become a substantial investment that needs to be weighed against the total amount of funds to be invested. However, if substantial sums are to be invested in advertising, for example, obtaining the services of a good advertising agency can be an investment that achieves high returns.

In sum. Marketing is an accepted activity for physicians and medical groups to engage in; however, many physicians are opposed to it. Physicians want to avoid the view that they are competing against other physicians. Physicians are also concerned that competition will cause the quality of care to deteriorate. Overcoming these sources of resistance might require careful and steady attention from hospital administrators to ensure that their relationship with a medical group is optimized.

Organizational Development

The value of a strategy also depends on the ability of a medical group to implement it. The best strategy can fail if the medical group involved is not able to implement its tactics. There are six variables medical groups and hospital administrators must attend to to implement a medical group's marketing strategy.

Structure

Structure means developing a formal organization for a medical group, including the promulgation of operating policies and procedures. It must be clear who is responsible for what and how tasks will be divided up. It must also be clear how individuals will be held accountable and by whom. A tightly designed structure might, in the beginning, be preferred over a loose one to ensure all physicians and staff acknowledge the rigorous formalized control. It might then become more informal as time passes and medical group members learn to appreciate the importance of compliance.

Hospital administrators should be certain that medical group members work through difficult-to-resolve issues that are often entangled with feelings about power and status. Hospital administrators might need to patiently coach physicians and staff and steadily advocate the resolution of these rather formal organizational considerations to resolve these anxiety-ridden elements of work life.

Shared Values

Shared values are the concepts and beliefs that members of the medical group hold in common. These values provide standards by which work can be measured, and they prescribe appropriate working relationships between individual medical group members. They also indicate what behavior is to be controlled and how. They point to the human qualities desired in medical group members, and they govern how members are to interact with the operating environment.

Hospital administrators must take the time to get to know the culture of medical groups they work with and avoid too quick of an appraisal, which, because of the more businesslike culture of the hospital, can lead to the condemnation of a medical group's unbusinesslike ways. Hospital administrators must appreciate that the culture that exists has been carefully developed over an extended period of time in what amounts to, at times, unconscious group processes aimed at relieving anxieties about working with each other, with patients, and in the marketplace. Deep-seated conflict will arise around any condemnation of or efforts to surreptitiously change the culture. In sum, care and respect must be paid when dealing with sensitive matters of medical group culture.

Management Style

Management style refers to how the medical group's managers, leaders, and physicians relate to employees, patients, and the public. Superior practices are managed by people who are effective at keeping employees and staff working on their tasks while not ignoring the human side of the enterprise. The impact of good or bad management styles and methods cannot be underestimated. A medical group can significantly enhance its effectiveness by effective leadership, and even the best of groups can be crippled by leadership that becomes political, absent, autocratic, self-centered, and unilateral.

Hospital administrators must gain a clear understanding of the leadership styles used by a medical group's physicians and nonphysician managers. Physicians in particular are often hard to understand when they assume leadership roles that they have not been educated to handle. They often rely on a process of piecing together a leadership style that meets their unique needs to minimize anxiety while providing enough direction for the medical group. Hospital administrators, if patient, can eventually offer yet another locus of leadership, which medical groups that are unhappy with their current leadership might welcome.

Staff

Staff must possess skills consistent with the elements of the medical group's marketing strategy, mix, and tactics. Employees must be trained to relate to patients and the public effectively, and they must be properly trained to deliver services. Being prepared to offer friendly, efficient, and effective service is critical for competitive success in the 1990s, as has been illustrated by the steadily increasing attention many large service organizations and hospitals are giving to guest relations training programs. Hospital administrators can support the development of these skills via hospital training programs.

Systems

Medical group information, accounting, budgeting, operating, quality assurance, and performance measurement systems must be designed with the group's strategy and tactics in mind. For the medical group to understand what is happening and why, the systems must be consistent with the group's overall purpose. For example, lack of good accounting and management information systems can make efforts to achieve a low-cost, high-quality position difficult.

Hospital administrators can bring to bear the expertise of staff who specialize in system design and development. Computing specialists, system and management analysts, management engineers, and internal auditors can all contribute to improving practice business systems and help the medical group win success in the marketplace.

Participation

Smooth implementation of change is facilitated if all practice staff are kept informed. Whenever possible, participation should be encouraged. Staff and physicians not directly involved in planning have valuable ideas and can offer information that will assist those developing the plans. Opportunities to participate meaningfully are positively experienced by those who are critical to making the changes work but are also customarily left out. Sincerity is the key to participation. Arranging structured meetings that permit only one-way communication under the guise of participation will not be experienced as a legitimate opportunity to participate. Developing participation involves a commitment to communicate planning progress to others and to listen to their ideas and thoughts. As a result, they feel better about themselves, the medical group, and its leadership. Problems that are so often encountered when implementing change are minimized by simply permitting participation. Hospital administrators should encourage participation by modeling the desired behavior through letting as many members of the medical group participate as is prudent.

Conclusion

Hospitals and medical groups can find many areas where a collaborative approach to planning and marketing will yield win-win outcomes. This chapter has focused attention on many of these areas in the hope that the discussion will help to guide those exploring hospital-physician networking.

6

LEGAL ISSUES FOR
HOSPITAL-PHYSICIAN NETWORKING

The growing interest of health care providers in forming new alliances and joint ventures has attracted the attention of Congress, the Department of Justice, and many state attorneys general. Hospital administrators and physicians are well advised to consult with legal counsel before starting negotiations to develop a physician network. Many states have legal doctrines that prohibit lay persons and corporations from employing or contracting with physicians for medical services; in the minds of legislators, such relationships might interfere with the physician-patient relationship.

This chapter focuses on three legal issues involved in hospital-physician networking arrangements: (1) fraud and abuse, (2) alternative organizational structures, and (3) antitrust activity and restraint of trade. The history of fraud and abuse relative to physicians and hospitals and safe harbor regulations that deal with this issue are examined. The chapter continues by describing the problems PHOs have in finding a corporate structure that meets their needs and will pass muster with the regulators. The chapter concludes by looking at how networking is being closely monitored for antitrust and restraint of trade violations.

Fraud and Abuse

Concern for fraud and abuse began with the Medicare and Medicaid programs. The Medicare and Medicaid Fraud and Abuse Statute defines fraudulent activity. It is illegal for an individual or legal entity to file false claims, to solicit or receive remuneration in return for patient referrals, or to offer or pay remuneration to invite referrals. Violations are premised on the willful or knowing solicitation, offer, payment, or receipt of "any remuneration" in return for or to induce the referral of a patient whose health care costs are paid at least in part by Medicare or Medicaid. The statute also contains criminal penalties, including fines up to $25,000, imprisonment up to five years, or both, and civil penalties up to $2,000 per violation plus an assessment against violators of up to twice the amount of the claims affected.[1] The Statute is enforced by the U.S. Department of Justice, which has authority to initiate criminal proceedings, and the Office of Inspector General (OIG) of the Department of Health and Human Services (DHHS). The OIG can impose civil penalties and expel violators from the Medicare and Medicaid programs.

During the early years of Medicare and Medicaid, these enforcement agencies focused on identifying and apprehending physicians and other providers who were defrauding these entitlement programs by submitting false claims for payment. Some physicians believed an audit was unlikely and found it tempting to submit claims for patients who either did not exist or for services not rendered. The rationale often given by the violators was that the programs did not provide sufficient reimbursement and that they were, therefore, justified in gaining the additional payments.

More recently, the development of joint business ventures between physicians, private investors, and hospitals has expanded the role of the regulators. In addition to watching for fraudulent claims submission, they are also now looking for business ventures that encourage the profitable utilization of perhaps unnecessary services by providing financial incentives to providers to prescribe the services.

There are two common scenarios. The first involves a physician who participates in the ownership of an ancillary service organization to which he or she sends patients for service. An example of this scenario is a neurologist who is part owner of a stand-alone imaging center. The second involves an agreement that rewards a physician for referring patients for service. An example of this is a reference laboratory that provides incentives for physicians' referrals. The incentives might include anything from cash payments to travel benefits, dinners, and gifts. Hospitals are also in a position to direct patients to vendors of outside goods and services, as might be the case in the purchase of durable medical equipment or follow-up home care and, as a result, are also being subjected to scrutiny.

The statute's intent is to avoid these types of abuses, and it is note-worthy that the statute is written in broad language that permits many physician ventures and business arrangements to be held suspect. Legitimate confusion over which types of practices are forbidden has led Congress and the DHHS to provide additional guidance through statutory and regulatory "safe harbors." Safe harbors explain conduct that does not violate the statute.

The OIG, during the summer of 1991, issued its long-awaited regulations defining safe harbors, which guide investment and involvement in networking. The following is a description of how the regulations affect the development of hospital-physician networks.

Investment in Small Business Entities

The most important venture opportunity that the regulations address is one where hospitals or physicians (or persons in a position to refer patients) have an ownership position in the business receiving the referrals. The safe harbor permits referrals when no more than a 40 percent interest is held by investors who are in a position to make or influence referrals to the provider. A good example of this type of situation involves the joint ownership of a pharmacy by a hospital and physicians located in a medical office building adjacent to the hospital. Both parties are in a position to influence where patients fill their prescriptions. In this case, outside investors must possess 60 percent ownership.

The other condition of this safe harbor is that no more than 40 percent of the provider's business can come from investors. This safe harbor is aimed at situations where a physician or medical group only owns a 25 percent interest but refers 75 percent of the business. An example is a surgeon's involvement with an outpatient surgery center.

Safe harbor regulations also more clearly define what is considered to be fraudulent behavior. These situations include

- investment arrangements in which investors are chosen because they are in a position to make referrals,
- arrangements in which investors are encouraged to maintain a certain level of referrals and are required to divest themselves of their investment if referrals are curtailed for any reason, and
- arrangements in which physician-investors commit substantial amounts of capital or in which the risk to the physician-investor is inordinately small in relation to the expected or actual returns.

An example of an arrangement that violates these rules is one in which a referring physician receives remuneration in the form of a consulting or advisory fee but performs little if any work to earn the remuneration. This type of arrangement is understood to be a mechanism to pay the referring physician for referrals.

Space Rental Agreements

Safe harbor regulations also regulate the practice of hospitals leasing space in a hospital-owned medical office building to physicians on their medical staffs. The OIG found physicians were being provided low-cost leases as a form of compensation for their referrals to their hospital. Safe harbor regulations now require that a signed lease of at least one-year duration be executed and that the rent be assessed at fair market value. Equipment rental arrangements must meet similar criteria to pass the safe harbor test.

Management Services Contracts

These types of arrangements are permitted as long as they meet the same fair-market-value requirements as those for space and equipment rental. Additionally, the service provided cannot promote a business arrangement between the parties. An example is a hospital providing management services to a medical group and using the relationship to promote the use of the hospital's services.

Physician Referral Services

Many hospitals have found a physician referral service to be an effective way to draw patients to their hospital. Traditionally, these services have only been provided to members of the hospital's medical staff. These services must now also meet safe harbor regulations. The services must be open to all potentially interested physicians. Charges for the services must be the same for all participants, and patients must be made aware of the criteria that govern physician involvement such as that many of the physicians involved are on the medical staff of the hospital.

Sale of Physician Practices

The safe harbor regulation for the sale of physician practices applies only to a sale between physicians. In this case the selling practitioners must sever their relationship with the practice within one year of the sale. This proviso prevents an arrangement where a selling physician profits from continuing to refer patients to the buyers.

The OIG regulations specifically state that this safe harbor is not meant to include hospital purchases of physician practices where the physician becomes a member of the hospital's medical staff. As a result, hospitals need to take special precautions in structuring acquisitions of medical practices to avoid scrutiny that the hospital is acquiring a medical practice to gain or maintain referrals. Some hospitals have tried to avoid scrutiny by stating in their buyout agreement that the physicians are free to send or admit their patients to any hospital they choose. The following is an example of such a statement:

> The terms and conditions of this agreement have not been offered for the purpose of requiring or inducing referrals or the utilization of hospital X. Physicians in medical group Y shall have complete discretion in selecting the site for their inpatient or outpatient hospital and diagnostic services.

It is interesting to note that the OIG, while expressing concern about physician-physician ventures, does not seem to be as concerned about potential abuses in physician-hospital arrangements. Perhaps their reasoning is that physician-hospital relationships do not necessarily lead to financial incentives for physicians. The hospital does not pay physicians for their referrals. A physician, as a member of the medical staff, will admit or refer his or her patients to the hospital anyway regardless of whether further inducements are offered. The scenario that the OIG is concerned about, however, is a hospital buying a practice that has members who were not previously on the hospital's medical staff. Such a purchase suggests that the hospital is buying admissions and referrals.

Another problem area occurs when a hospital is invited into a relationship because of financial need on the part of a physician or medical group. The practice might be seen to be obligated to the hospital for the bailout. It seems reasonable to expect that the physicians would feel uncomfortable with continuing to refer patients to a competing hospital

The OIG has also announced that more rulings are forthcoming. The indications are that they will provide safe harbor regulations for physician-physician and hospital-physician ventures such as physicians referring their patients to an organization where they also provide the service. An example is an orthopedic surgeon referring a patient to an investor-owned outpatient surgical care center where the surgeon is also an owner. Additionally, hospital payment arrangements that cover some types of physician expenses, such as for physician recruitment and professional liability insurance, are also items that might be addressed by future rulings.

In sum, the OIG's approach appears to be one of providing safe harbors only for investments or arrangements that can be clearly understood to avoid conflicts of interests. However, given the nature of legalistic maneuvers, some physicians and hospital administrators might react not by focusing on the intent of the safe harbors but rather by preferring to walk a legal tightrope by minimally and legalistically complying with the guidelines. This approach, combined with the rapid pace of venture development, can well become costly for physicians and hospital administrators who assume that their arrangements are safe from current or new regulations that forbid the practices. Divestiture can become expensive remediation.

Alternatives for Structuring Hospital-Physician Relationships

The idea of hospitals helping physicians to get organized is intimidating; however, it is to the advantage of hospitals to ensure they do. If hospital administrators are to take the lead in responding to the demands for cost controls, higher quality, and comprehensive services, they need their physicians to work with them.

Hospitals and physicians who attempt to go it alone and independently deal with the changing health care delivery and finance system lose the benefit of synergy, which reduces redundancy and inefficiency. A better strategy is for hospitals and physicians to collaborate to garner better contracts, improve their risk exposure, and reduce inefficiencies in their delivery of care. However, working together requires a common organizational structure to combine leadership and to set common direction. The appropriate legal structure is also important from a reimbursement standpoint. Collections from third parties can be optimized by carefully structuring who bills for what.

There are three principal forms of hospital-physician organizational arrangements: hospital employment of physicians, medical foundation, and management services organizations (MSOs).

Employment of Physicians

The most straightforward approach for hospitals to take in creating a formal link with physicians is to employ them. As an employee, a physician's clinical and administrative activity is under the control of the hospital's management structure. The most common scenario for this approach is for the hospital to hire a solo practitioner or members of a medical group. Physicians who are nearing retirement and anticipate having difficulty finding someone to buy their practices might be particularly receptive. Hospital administrators might be interested because they want the physician's location and patient base to remain connected with their hospital. Another common situation is new physicians just going into practice who do not want to invest in starting their own practices to become hospital employees and give the hospital the risk of developing their practices.

It is recommended that the hospital execute an employment agreement. Appendix 6.1 is an example of a physician employment contract.

Employment agreements should cover the following points:

1. *Purpose and employment.* This section defines the purpose of the agreement and establishes the parties to the agreement, the hospital (Employer), and the physician (Employee).

2. *Term.* Establishing the term of employment is important. The hospital might want the flexibility of annual terms in the event the physician does not perform satisfactorily. However, hospital administrators must appreciate that this arrangement presents physicians with a new experience. As a result, their response might be uncertain. Another situation where this flexibility is helpful is where a hospital is gambling that a new medical office or clinic will attract the needed business. A short-term lease and employment agreement allows the hospital to escape major losses.

3. *Duties.* This is the most important section of the agreement. The hospital should not hesitate to delineate the duties and responsibilities of the physician. If the hospital expects the physician to participate in quality assurance and utilization review or to serve in a management capacity, the duties should be listed. Appendix 6.1, for example, specifies that the physician is to split his or her time between several clinics. The days and hours must be specified.

4. *Performance.* This section imposes restrictions on the physician in terms of services provided or outside activities. A religious hospital might, for example, prohibit the delivery of services that are not consistent with its beliefs. Any outside practice may also be ruled out.

5. *Compensation and benefits.* Several sections might be needed to define the physician's salary and benefits. The primary consideration for the hospital is that the physician has been accustomed to a certain level of salary and benefits that he or she will not want to see interrupted or decreased. There are also other expenses physicians incur, such as professional insurance, license costs, medical society dues, and continuing education courses, that should be addressed.

6. *Facilities, files, and records.* The agreement should define the space the physician will work in. In many cases, the hospital offers to employ the physician and lease his or her current office for him or her to use. This again offers the hospital the flexibility of terminating the relationship by not owning a clinic. A physician's patient files and records should become the property of the hospital. As in Appendix 6.1, the hospital might choose to allow the physician

to take his or her patient records should he or she terminate the employment arrangement and enter or return to private practice.

7. *Ability to perform.* The agreement should include a section to cover the possibility that the physician is unable to perform his or her duties due to medical problems. Compensation during a disability period and the process for determining the ability to return to work should be specified. This is extremely important to the hospital due to the difficulty in finding a temporary replacement physician.

8. *Termination.* The agreement should define the causes for terminating a physician. The usual causes are loss of licensure, loss of hospital staff privileges, arrest, and displinary action by a medical review organization. The hospital might also want to impose other guidelines more specific to the employment arrangement.

In sum, employing physicians is not as casy as executing a purchasing contract. The hospital administrator should remember that the physician is going to find the new arrangement difficult. He or she is very likely used to a great deal of autonomy that has included the length of vacations and how office operations and staff are managed. The physician, by becoming a part of a much larger organization, has to learn to share authority and comply with directives from senior management who might not always anticipate how physicians think or work.

Medical Foundation Models of Organization

Employing physicians and using them to staff hospital-owned clinics sounds like the ultimate hospital-physician integration. Unfortunately, not every physician is ready to give up his or her autonomy and financial independence to go to work for a hospital. Physicians in larger group practices see themselves in a stronger position as compared to their solo practice and small group practice colleagues. However, while they might not be willing to throw in the towel on their independence, they are often willing to align themselves with a hospital to achieve some of the joint strategic advantages mentioned in Chapter 5.

One organizational model that permits this type of hospital-physician integration is the medical foundation model (see Figure 6.1). This model entails the hospital and physicians creating a 501(c)(3) tax-exempt nonprofit foundation to do the following:

- Purchase all the assets of the physicians involved in the venture
- Employ the nonphysician staff of the physicians involved

Figure 6.1 Medical Foundation Model

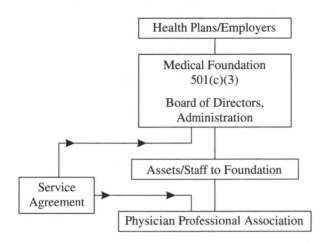

- Contract with the physician's professional corporation for the provision of physician patient services

The foundation is a freestanding, tax-exempt legal entity that owns all the assets needed to provide patient services. These assets usually include medical office buildings, physician patient accounts receivable, and equipment and furniture. The physicians form a professional association or partnership to contract with the foundation to provide them a place to practice and a salary.

This model addresses a number of issues that plague larger group practices.

1. Existing medical groups often experience the problem of the older founding physicians requiring an expensive buyout. This arrangement makes a buyin for the new younger physician expensive. The physician contract for services solves this problem as there is no financial interest in the foundation. Their only interest is in their compensation arrangement, which is negotiated within the physician association. There is no physician equity to be bought out by new physicians.

2. The foundation provides the capital needed to purchase equipment or to build facilities.

3. The foundation provides the administrative and support staff and is responsible for developing benefit and retirement plans.

4. The foundation contracts with managed care plans and employers for hospital and physician services, thereby sharing risk with the physician organization.

5. The foundation's organizational structure requires joint quality and utilization review of both hospital and physician services.

The ownership of the foundation is important. In some cases the hospital creates it and is the sole member of it. In others, the effort includes physicians. If the goal is to promote cooperation, the joint board makeup is more appropriate. However, regardless of how it is structured, the hospital will want to have physician representation on the board. Often, lay members of the community are also invited to serve on the board.

Several legal conditions must be met when establishing a foundation. First, the structure must qualify for 501(c)(3) status.[2] The foundation must have a charitable or educational aspect to its mission. Foundations associated with large group practices invariably provide a site for student and house staff education and training, patient education, and research programs. Secondly, the foundation must also be able to show that its relationship with its physicians will not result in private inurement. This is where lay board membership helps to dilute physician participation. Another issue is how pension plans are dealt with between the foundation and the physician association. Due to their close association, the threat exists that the IRS might view separate plans for the physicians and the foundation staff as one. Questions can also arise over credentialing and peer review. It should be clear who is to perform these functions, the foundation or the physician association. It should also be clear for the foundation how malpractice insurance is covered between the hospital and the physician association.

In sum, it is important that the parties maintain an arm's length relationship when putting this type of venture together. The appearance of becoming aligned legal entities that are not able to keep business transactions separate could eventually lead to federal and state intervention.

The Management Service Organization

Another innovative approach to hospital-physician relations is the development of MSOs. MSOs (Figure 6.2) are patterned after medical staff–hospital plans (MeSHs). MeSHs are joint ventures created by a hospital and physicians to enter into risk-sharing contracts with payers covering both inpatient and physician services.

In contrast, MSOs can be either wholly owned subsidiaries of hospitals or hospital-physician joint ventures. Large MSOs have the administrative

Figure 6.2 The Management Service Organization Model

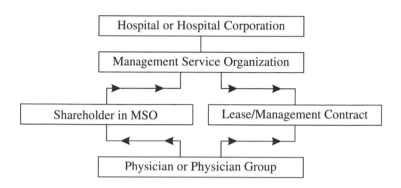

and support staff and equipment necessary to operate a medical practice or an IPA. The MSO leases its staff and equipment to the practice or IPA in a turnkey fashion at a set fee or as a percentage of the contractee's business. The medical practice or IPA remains the decision maker for services and retains ownership of the practice and patient medical records. The MSO simply serves as a management company that offers staff and equipment to physicians for a fee. This kind of arrangement provides small- to medium-size medical groups with desired practice independence while enabling them to access administrative expertise and business equipment without capital outlay. Management service organization services can also include marketing, computerized patient billing, and clinic management. These organizations differ from foundations in that the physicians remain independent both in terms of practice decisions and ownership. The same legal uncertainties that concern the foundation model are also present with the MSO. The arrangements must be free of fraud and abuse. Inurement issues must be avoided.

Antitrust Concerns

In addition to being concerned about fraud and abuse and illegal organizational structures, regulators are also concerned about the antitrust aspect of hospital-physician relationships. Like most other industries, the health care industry produces competition between its providers, particularly in urban areas. Government has not historically been greatly concerned with either price fixing or restraint of trade activity in health care because of the large number of physicians and hospitals involved. However, the new relationship-building activities of hospitals and physicians is beginning to focus increasing attention on activities that threaten to reduce competition and lead to illegal price setting or, perhaps more accurately, reimbursement setting.

The development of health care corporations that encompass hospitals, physician practices, and other service organizations that consolidate the delivery of services and channel them into a more efficient process promises to reduce costs. However, there is evidence that some alliances have been formed for the purposes of maintaining price levels in a community to countervail pressure from managed care plans as they try to negotiate lower costs. This is particularly true in small communities where there is one hospital and a small cadre of physicians. This movement therefore opposes the growth of managed care organizations and the government's movement via DRGs and RBRVS toward a payer pricing system.

The dilemma for regulators is whether to restrict this activity in the name of the restriction of trade or to allow it in the name of the public good. Proponents of alliances used for price negotiation argue that collaboration is needed because large purchasers have an unfair advantage when negotiating reimbursement. They argue that joint development activities are good for the community and cost effective and that the development of new facilities, physicians, and technology enhances the availability of efficient quality services to a community.

However, as the threat of large PHOs looms on the horizon, access to a choice of providers by the public has also become an issue. As hospitals move to consolidate their medical staffs both by specialty and location, they establish geographic boundaries for their target service. Once control of the service area is established, it becomes difficult for other hospitals to compete in the same area. The public is then left with, for all practical purposes, receiving care from one health care delivery organization. This possibility leads to the conjecture that, in the future, people living in urban areas might choose where to live relative to established health care system territories, as they now do relative to townships, school and water districts, and voting precincts.

In sum, public policymakers face a difficult dilemma. They must decide if competition in the health care industry tends to produce the lowest costs and maximum quality and access. Arguments are now surfacing that the solution, in lieu of a free market, is to increase government regulation and control. Proponents argue that states should regulate the activities of health care providers and purchasers to achieve access for all, low cost, freedom of choice, and high quality—an outcome surely to be resisted by most health care delivery participants.

Conclusion

The economics and politics of health care are pushing providers to the edge of testing what is legal as they struggle to maintain the control of their industry. The government is beginning to realize that part of the solution to the rise in health care costs is the integration of the provider arena to eliminate duplication and take advantage of economies of scale. The question that must now be answered is what latitude will be given to hospitals and physicians to work together to contribute to the solution.

Appendix 6.1
Example of a Physician Employment Agreement

Saint Mary's Hospital: Employment Agreement

This agreement is made April 1, 1991, between Saint Mary's Hospital [all names are fictitious], a Minnesota nonprofit corporation, Employer, and John R. Smith, M.D., Physician.

THE PARTIES AGREE AS FOLLOWS:

1. *Purpose and employment.* The purpose of this agreement is to define the relationship between Employer, as an employer, and Physician, as an employee of Employer. By executing this agreement, Employer employees Physician, and Physician accepts employment by Employer, on the terms and conditions set forth in this agreement.

2. *Term.* The term of this agreement shall commence on the date of the agreement and shall terminate on December 31, 1993, or on the effective date of termination of employment as provided in this agreement. Notwithstanding the above, if Employer is unable to engage a replacement physician, Physician's employment shall be extended until June 30, 1994, on terms and conditions to which the parties may mutually agree.

3. *Duties.* Physician shall practice medicine exclusively and solely as an employee of Employer and shall devote his/her entire professional time to the affairs of Employer. Physician shall practice at the medical clinics located in the cities of Walnut Grove and Worth, Minnesota.

4. *Performance.* Physician agrees as follows:

a. Physician shall devote all necessary time and Physician's best efforts in the performance of his/her duties as a licensed physician for Employer in accordance with the highest ethical duties as are assigned to Physician from time to time by Employer.

b. Physician shall maintain a membership on the medical staff with full clinical privileges at the hospitals in the area where the medical clinics are located.

c. Unless Employer otherwise agrees, Physician shall practice medicine full time at the medical clinics. For the purposes of this agreement, the practice of full-time medicine shall mean that the Physician shall be available at the clinic offices two half days each week at the Walnut Grove clinic and two half days and three full days at the Worth clinic.

d. Physician shall not perform any procedures that are inconsistent with the Catholic philosophy and identity as well as the Ethical and Religious Directives for Catholic Health Care Facilitates as published by the Catholic Health Association.

5. *Compensation.* For the services Physician rendered in any capacity under this agreement, Employer shall pay Physician an annual salary of $75,000, payable twice a month. If a replacement physician is found to cover the clinic hours at the Walnut Grove clinic, Physician's compensation shall be adjusted to 80 percent of this full-time rate, unless Physician's hours at the Worth clinic are increased.

6. *Benefits.* In addition to the compensation paid to Physician, Employer shall provide Physician with the same benefits as Physician was provided prior to Physician's employment.

7. *Expenses.* Employer recognizes that Physician will incur, from time to time, for Employer's benefit and in performance of Physician's practice, various expenses; and Employer agrees to pay directly, to advance sums to Physician to be used for expenses, or to reimburse Physician for expenses for the following items:

a. Professional liability (malpractice) insurance, provided that after the termination of employment, Physician shall be responsible for his/her own "tail" insurance.

b. Professional license fees, dues, and memberships not to exceed $500 per year

c. Professional convention and meeting expenses and continuing professional education expenses not to exceed $3,000 per year

8. *Working facilities.* Employer shall provide and maintain the facilities, equipment, and supplies it deems are necessary for Physician's performance of professional duties under this agreement. Employer shall provide Physician with an office, books, and stenographic and technical help.

9. *Files and records.* All case records, case histories, x-ray films, and regular files concerning patients of Employer, including, without limitation, patients consulted, interviewed, or treated by Physician during the term of this agreement, shall belong to and remain the property of Employer. On the termination of employment, Physician shall have the privilege, on the presentation of a written direction from each patient within one year after the termination, of reproducing, at Physician's own expense, any of Employer's files or records maintained for that patient during Physician's employment with Employer.

10. *Vacation and leave.* During each annual period, the first commencing on the date of employment and terminating on the last day of the twelfth month after that date, Physician shall be entitled to

a. a vacation leave of three weeks and

b. a leave to attend programs of continuing medical education and professional organizations of one week.

11. *Disability.* During the term of this agreement, if Physician is disabled, Physician shall receive 100 percent of his/her compensation for the first month of the disability and 50 percent of the compensation for the next three months. For the purpose of this paragraph, *disabled* or *disability* shall mean the physical or mental inability, as a result of illness, disease, or accident, to carry on the practice of medicine from day to day, efficiently and competently. Whether or not Physician is disabled under this agreement will be a question of fact to be decided according to accepted medical standards by a disinterested and competent physician selected by Employer. In determining periods of disability, periods of disability shall be counted as one disability if Physician has not returned to work for at least one month between such periods of disability.

12. *Termination.* Employer shall have the right to terminate this agreement immediately, on written notice to Physician, for any of the following reasons:

a. Revocation or suspension of Physician's license to practice in this state

b. Resignation by Physician from any professional organization while under threat of disciplinary action

c. Conviction of any crime punishable as a felony, gross misdemeanor, or a criminal offense involving moral turpitude or immoral conduct

d. Willful contravention of professional ethics or willful violation of any of the terms of this agreement

e. Failure of Physician to practice full time, as defined in this agreement, within the Walnut Grove, Minnesota area

   f. Revocation, suspension, qualification, restriction, limitation, or con-
   ditioning of clinical privileges as a member of the medical staff of
   any hospital at which Physician had established privileges

   13. *Binding effect.* This agreement shall be binding on the parties to
it and on their legal representatives, successors, and assigns.

   14. *Applicable law.* This agreement shall be governed for all purposes
under the laws of the State of Minnesota. If any provision of this Agreement
is declared null and void, that provision shall be deemed severed from this
agreement, which shall otherwise remain in full force and effect.

   15. *Noncompetition.* Physician agrees that for a period of four years
after the commencement date of his/her employment, he/she will not practice
medicine within a radius of 50 miles of the City of Walnut Grove, Minnesota,
except as an employee of Employer.

   16. *Assignment.* Physician's rights and benefits under this agreement
are personal to Physician, and no such right or benefit shall be subject to
voluntary or involuntary alienation, assignment, or transfer.

   17. *Entire agreement.* This agreement supersedes all other agreements
previously made by the parties relating to the subject matter. There are no
other understandings or agreements.

   18. *Nonwaiver.* No delay or failure by either party to exercise any
right under this agreement or no partial or single exercise of the right shall
constitute a waiver of that or any other right.

   19. *Notice.* Any notice to be delivered under this agreement shall be
given in writing and delivered, personally or by certified mail, addressed to
Employer or Physician at their last known addresses.

   IN WITNESS WHEREOF, the parties have executed this agreement
on the day and year first written above.

Physician: Employer:

                                    SAINT MARY'S HOSPITAL
_____
John R. Smith, M.D.

                                    By _____
                                       Peter J. Jones
                                       President

Notes

1. Social Security Act § 1320a(7)(b).
2. I.R.C. 501(c)(3).

7

Assessing the Leadership Politics of Medical Groups

Medical groups are composed of a mix of personnel, some of whom are among the most highly trained and educated of professionals. This rich mixture of diversity is a critical factor in how the members of a medical group relate to each other and manage the group. This chapter provides hospital administrators critically important information about how physicians work and suggestions about how best to work with and sometimes manage them. The content of the chapter facilitates assessing both how well a medical group is managed and how it should be managed to promote effectiveness should a formal relationship be desirable.

In particular this chapter focuses on the dominant influence of physicians who own and operate medical groups. Their personalities result in a variety of supervisory and leadership styles that dominate group dynamics. To be discussed first is the impact of their personalities on interpersonal relations and leadership styles. The chapter concludes with an examination of how these hard-to-control personality variables can be, in part, managed through organizational structure as represented by bylaws, goals and objectives, and policies and procedures.

Physicians Learn Their Behavior

Physicians are intelligent, well-educated people who provide highly personal health care services. Physicians are expected to be sensitive to patients' needs and are not expected to make mistakes; they must correctly diagnose and treat their patients. At the same time, physicians have experienced the same developmental problems we have all had to face from infancy to adulthood, and despite their intellectual gifts, they have limitations as well. In sum, physicians are imperfect human beings who feel they must achieve perfection in their work. These profoundly conflicted expectations lead to reliance on social and psychological defenses such as the physician's cloak of unquestionable (and usually not understandable) expertise, the denial of imperfections, and the depersonalization of their patients. These interpersonal defenses in the practice of medicine are also consistent with the following psychological analysis of leadership styles.

Physician executives believe that, as in the practice of medicine, they must impose their will on decision making, others, and events. These tendencies lead to autocratic or dictatorial, manipulative or pseudodemocratic, authoritarian, paternalistic, and task-oriented leadership styles. These typical leadership styles share the need to control the situation and others and are associated with positive self-feelings of being powerful and superior. The physician executive might feel he or she is the only person capable of making the right decisions. Opposition must be defeated. The pursuit of perfection and power can also be accompanied by narcissistic tendencies. The physician, as the caregiver in an indifferent organization, can feel unadmired, unappreciated, and not cared about as a human being and work toward being admired and liked by rewarding those who are willing to feed his or her narcissism. Ironically, this same individual might act insensitively, autocratically, and vindictively toward those who feed the narcissism and who, it is understood at an unconscious level, are inferior and do not deserve better treatment.

These types of feelings and actions have predictable effects on others. Peers and staff become passive and compliant. Resisters might be fired, ignored, or pressured to leave. New staff are hired in the belief that they will support the culture of narcissism. In the end, staff become the admiring and uncritical audience the physician executive desires, thereby becoming a group that reinforces the leadership style.

Less frequently, a physician executive might avoid dealing with problems and prefer to let others make the tough decisions. This type of leadership style can be labeled: laissez-faire, democratic, permissive, humanistic, and insecure. Consensus building might become the norm. Everyone must agree to avoid hurt feelings. Intractable problems loaded with conflicting points of view might go unresolved to everyone's detriment.

In sum, it must be appreciated that physicians who become leaders enter into a situation for which they have no or little education and training, and they end up relying on their own ingenuity, perhaps a limited amount of reading, a lot of listening to and observation of role models, and, in the final analysis, their personalities to develop their leadership style. The development of these organic leadership styles can be better understood by reviewing the research of T. Alan Jensen.

Jensen performed a study involving 45 two-hour interviews of physician executives.[1] The interpretation of the interview data led him to develop a matrix of five physician executive leadership styles: (1) the practice physician executive, (2) the profession physician executive, (3) the self physician executive, (4) the organization physician executive, and (5) the syntonic physician executive. These five leadership patterns include specific philosophies toward medical organizations, specific approaches toward the task structure, specific approaches toward external groups, and specific image management concerns (see Table 7.1). Jensen concluded physician executives vacillate between the more balanced (syntonic) leadership style, which takes into consideration aspects of the other four leadership patterns, and the four less desirable leadership patterns. This classification scheme provides hospital administrators a way of understanding physician executive behavior. However, as pointed out, this classification scheme does not explain why physicians act these ways. To gain a better understanding of why, a psychological view of physician executives follows.

The Psychodynamics of Physician Executive Leadership Styles

Understanding human behavior is an admittedly complex and incomplete science. There are many different ways to understand what motivates people. The method presented here relies on a reasonably complete model of human behavior (Figure 7.1). The model is explained in jargon-free terms and possesses considerable explanatory power. In sum, even though the model's content is psychological and therefore possibly unfamiliar turf for managers, it is accessible and can benefit those who work with physicians.

Figure 7.1 depicts a psychodynamic model of human behavior under stress.[2] The model is especially useful for understanding the motivations of leaders who experience stress originating from both internal and external sources. The explanation of the model is followed by a discussion of its implications for understanding physician executive leadership styles.

Stress

Stress is defined as threatening events. Being disciplined or disapproved of and driving home on icy streets are stressful. Encountering resistance and rejection is stressful. The experience of an event as stressful (threatening to one's self) leads to feelings of anxiety that we all prefer to avoid.

Table 7.1 Five Physician Executive Leadership Styles

	Practice Physician	Profession Physician	Self Physician	Organization Physician	Syntonic Physician
Philosophy toward organization	Rational problem solving the best way to manage Humanistic attitude toward others Concerned with stability, cooperation, and harmony	Organization should provide stable and supportive structure that supports patient care Organizational norms do not apply to physicians seeking excellence and scientific discovery Health care organizations do not need to conform to social norms because of their mission	Organization is a battlefield for getting one's way Victories and defeats are only temporary; there will be more important battles to be waged	Organization can achieve ends through scientific management and rational structuring of the organization Team approach stressed where everyone is expected to contribute Advocate of organizational balance, no area outgrows others	Organizations need leaders who will take risks and make enemies Organizations need leaders who project the future Organizations should inspire others to excel, to assume leadership roles, and to work hard
Approach to task accomplishment	Funding provided based on demonstrated need Belief that persistence and pressure combined with rational argument will bring desired outcome	Direct assumption of responsibility, provides leadership and models excellence Other physicians and staff are expected to get work done in a professional manner	Control of all work and everyone desired Must know what everyone is doing Must make all the decisions Will manipulate others to win	Separates personal and organizational responsibilities Willing to devote large amounts of time to making the organization succeed Advocate of participation by others	Willing to work hard and direct the work of others as needed, able to make tough decisions Willing to support others and accept individual and situational limitations Keeps others on task and resolves differences of opinion without feeling the need to take charge and control everything

Approach to external groups	External groups viewed as a patient care resource Cooperation with external groups desirable	Autonomy from external groups is stressed Others are expected to learn the organization is unique and its positions are right Cooperation is sought from other powerful groups	Adept at relating to others who control external groups Does not believe norms and desires of others apply Willing to aggress against external groups to fulfill aims	Favors competing in the external environment Organizational rules should be changed to permit competitive success Favors negotiated agreements to control unproductive competition	Permits open and direct exchanges and seeks dialogue Promotes solutions to conflicts by emphasizing interrelatedness
Image management	Image of physician artisan Organization should help physician skills	Strives to develop aristocratic image and to differentiate self from other physicians in terms of importance Will collaborate with others who are working on tasks judged to be desirable (scientific)	Image of happy warrior Battles seen as means of improving organization	This competitor develops an image of capitalist and entrepreneur Paves way for the success of others Hires outstanding performers to enhance competitive edge	Projects image of wisdom and balance Able to deal with stress, diversity, and multiple issues without becoming distressed

Source: Adapted with permission of the publisher from T. A. Jensen, "Physician Executive Leadership," *Medical Group Management,* September/October 1986, 25. Copyright 1986, Medical Group Management Association.

Figure 7.1 Psychodynamic Model of Executive Leadership

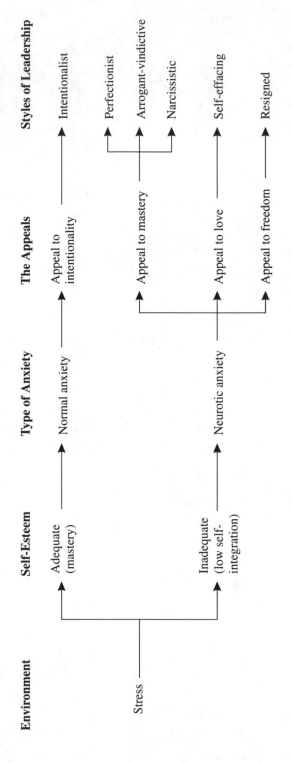

Source: Adapted, by permission of the publisher, from M. Diamond and S. Allcorn, "Psychological Barriers to Personal Responsibility," *Organizational Dynamics*, Spring 1984, 70, ©1984. American Management Association, New York. All rights reserved.

Self-Esteem

Self-esteem is defined as one's ability to cope with stress without losing self-confidence and self-integration. The interaction of stress and self-esteem leads either to feelings of normal anxiety, where self-confidence and self-integration are sustained, or neurotic anxiety, where self-confidence is lost and self-fragmentation occurs. The development of self-esteem starts at birth. An infant who feels insecure with a mother who is insensitive and unpredictable will develop a fragile, insecure, vulnerable sense of self that complicates successfully coping with stressful events and interpersonal relationships. Consequently, life can become filled with uncontrollable and unavoidable feelings of distress; therefore, the need arises for psychological defenses that are compulsively relied on to dispose of the anxiety.

Anxiety Levels

The model depicts a situation where adequate self-esteem permits the self-confident handling of a stressful event. Normal anxiety is experienced and the stressor does not become overly threatening. In contrast, where inadequate self-esteem exists, the same situation can be experienced as unmanageable and threatening and lead to the experience of neurotic anxiety. In the model, this neurotic anxiety results in three self-defensive tendencies that, in turn, form the basis for five leadership styles.

Responses to Anxiety

The model depicts normal anxiety as leading to the nondefensive appeal to intentionality. The three self-defensive tendencies, however, are responses loaded with compulsive needs to avoid feeling neurotic anxiety.[3] These responses, it is emphasized, are enduring responses that are worked out throughout life to deal with anxiety and might all be realized at one time or another, although one will be more frequent and constitute the basis of a leadership style.

The Appeal to Intentionality

The appeal to intentionality avoids disproportionate, compulsive, and inappropriate leadership behavior. This appeal, in contrast to those that follow, does not involve excessive reliance on psychological defenses. A genuine sense of self-esteem is maintained. Characteristic behaviors are nondefensive acceptance of criticism and feedback, self-reflection, appreciation of the thoughts and feelings of others, flexible and critical thinking, innovation, willingness to change, adherence to many aspects of rational decision-making processes, and awareness of the operating environment.

The Appeal to Mastery

The appeal to mastery is a tendency to feel everything must be mastered through willful domination and control. If the physician feels he or she is energetic enough, smart enough, manipulative enough, aggressive enough, and persistent enough, anything can be accomplished. These feelings have their origins in contempt for feelings of weakness and dependence that were very likely experienced early in life. The appeal to mastery requires an extensive investment in maintaining a powerful, nearly perfect self-image that is highly consistent with physician socialization. Should difficulties develop in maintaining the image, every effort is made to overcome the threat. That failing, the threat might be denied or rationalized. This self-image, as will be shown, implies contempt for others as it is others who must be bent to the physician's will.

The appeal to mastery leads to three leadership styles: perfectionistic, arrogant-vindictive, and narcissistic.

Perfectionistic style. Physicians who use this leadership style set nearly perfect standards for self-conduct and for what others think, feel, and do. The standards permit the physician to feel he or she is better than others, and as a result, they are rigidly adhered to. Additionally, implied in meeting the standards is that others will treat the physician as desired. Others must learn and meet the standards or risk being judged as deficient.

The perfectionistic leadership style has identifiable behavioral attributes. Among the more common and most easily identified are meticulous attention to detail and order, overpunctuality, careful dress and selection of words, high moral and ethical standards, and an excessively critical view of the behavior and work of others. These are attributes that are readily associated with physicians.

Arrogant-vindictive style. The physician who develops an arrogant-vindictive leadership style possesses arrogant self-pride and promotes competitive win-lose dynamics where he or she must win. Weakness, self-doubt, and dependence are abhorred. Anyone that gets in the way or injures his or her excessive pride must be defeated. This individual is capable of destructive rages and can be willing to take great risks to win.

This leader has easily identifiable patterns of behavior. This physician is competitive, arrogant, vindictive, and contemptuous of others (although it might be cloaked in civility). There is a desire to dominate, humiliate, and exploit others. The individual might think nothing of making excessive demands on others or violating accepted norms (rules do not apply to this superior person). Executive positions are often desired as a means of becoming powerful enough to defeat others. These types of behavior most likely arise for physician leaders when they encounter resistance to their ideas, hard-to-resolve conflict, personnel problems, and other types of situations that make them anxious.

Narcissistic style. The narcissistic physician leader's style is to appear competent and in control of one's self and the situation in the hope that he or she will be admired and trusted. This physician wants to be perceived as a great leader and seeks out those who reinforce the belief. The narcissistic physician leader also has identifiable behavior patterns. This individual seems loving, caring, and generous toward others to encourage their admiration. Physicians are often held in high esteem by many of those who work with them. This leader also often fails to recognize his or her limitations by making grand plans while paying little attention to details that will assure success.

The appeal to mastery can be briefly summarized. The physician executive who resorts to this appeal relies on all three leadership styles; however, one is expected to be more common. Traits associated with the appeal to mastery are (1) glorification and cultivation of everything that means or leads to power and mastery; (2) the need to excel and be superior; (3) readiness to manipulate and dominate others; (4) the pursuit of adoration, respect, or recognition; and (5) abhorrence for being compliant, appeasing, and dependent.

Physicians who must feel that they are in control of most situations most commonly rely on the appeal to mastery. As a result, professional managers who work with physicians can easily come to feel frustrated and anxious about how they are being treated. Regrettably, much of what the managers do and how they go about doing it will seem foreign to many physicians and therefore anxiety provoking. The predictable response to the anxiety-provoking behavior is a resort to some type of mastery. Fault in the manager's work, reports, and analyses might be rigorously sought out. He or she might become the focal point for unrelenting suspicion, denigration, and passive and active aggression. And last, the manager might be subjected to manipulations that encourage him or her to admire and like the physician.

The likelihood of exactly which type of behavior is acted out can tenuously be linked to the specialty of the physician. A dermatologist might well be much less aggressive and mastery oriented than, for example, a surgeon who, if crossed, might well become enraged and vindictive. In general and at the risk of oversimplifying, managers often find that physicians who do invasive procedures and who work close to life and death situations are generally more likely to vigorously pursue mastery (and when it comes to patient care, rightly so) than, say, family practitioners and internists. Some of the latter physicians might even possess some of the following behavioral tendencies.

The Appeal to Love

The appeal to love is a tendency to long for being protected and loved. This individual does not feel he or she is capable of mastery and might, in fact, abhor being masterful and in control. This tendency therefore is the opposite of the appeal to mastery. The person willingly subordinates himself or herself to others in an act of selfless devotion with the expectation of being loved and taken care of in return.

The appeal to love has a number of recognizable behaviors. Avoided are acting and feeling competent and confident. Self-esteem is low. The person is passive and low on assertion and might well feel inferior and contemptible. This person also (1) is noncompetitive and prefers to let others have their way, (2) avoids attracting attention to himself or herself, (3) abhors self-centered behavior, and (4) values loveable qualities such as unselfishness, goodness, generosity, humility, vulnerability, and sympathy. In return this "warm fuzzy" person hopes to be cared for and loved by others. The appeal to love becomes the self-effacing leadership style.

This type of behavior is encountered when a physician leader acts as though he or she is relatively ignorant and helpless and turns over virtually all administrative matters to a manager whom the physician feels is authoritative. This level of delegation, while flattering to the manager, must be appreciated for what it is. It is less a function of an acknowledgement of the manager's skills and more a function of how the physician feels about himself or herself. The manager must appreciate that he or she is being subjected to the appeal and therefore is expected to be caring.

The Appeal to Freedom

The appeal to freedom is a tendency to feel that conflicts and problems at work cannot be dealt with and to think that withdrawal from active participation is the only solution. Life without pain and problems is desired, which leads to a life with few strong feelings and little energy and risk taking. The person seeks inner peace by sacrificing active participation in life.

This appeal also results in identifiable behavior. The person holds few self-expectations and lacks the drive to set goals or accomplish work. The person prefers to be left alone and might appear to others to have become an onlooker to his or her own life. Similarly, the person seems detached from others and events. The essence of the appeal is that it frees the person from obligations and stress and becomes the resigned leadership style.

Physicians exhibit this behavior when they take the position that they just want to be left alone to practice medicine or perform research. This behavior might also be encountered when physician leaders find dealing with problems too tough and act to avoid them and conflict.

Self-Defensive Behavioral Tendencies: A Recapitulation

The three defensive behavioral tendencies and six leadership styles offer a readily understandable means of analyzing most physician executive behavior. It is also important to appreciate that the appeals represent mutually exclusive categories for classifying behavior in that it is not possible to realize (act out) more than one appeal at a time. A person cannot seek the appeal to mastery while simultaneously appealing to love (its opposite) or freedom, which avoids dealing with problems all together. However, conflicting thoughts and feelings can be held simultaneously, and changes in defensive behavior can be so rapid that they appear to be being acted out at the same time. Indeed, the nature of this conflict motivates compulsive behavior.

It is also important to appreciate that the three defensive tendencies and the intentional tendency include most of the behavior of physician leaders. Physicians might deal with a stressful situation, seek to control and dominate it, flee from it, or look to someone else to take care of it. It is also worth noting that the above discussion of the defensive tendencies complements Jenson's study of physician leadership styles.

Given that physicians might adopt many different and not always functional leadership styles, what can be done about the work-related dysfunctions that they create?

Strategies for Intervention

The appreciation thus far gained for the psychodynamic elements that underlie leadership styles should indicate no list of steps can be provided to deal effectively with psychologically defensive physician leadership styles. Rather, what is learned from the psychodynamic model is the need on the part of the physician executive to act out behavior in the pursuit of relief from feeling anxious. Directly challenging the behavior can be depended on to create more anxiety and perhaps a vindictive response or a greater need for admiration by a group specially developed to meet the needs (a "kitchen cabinet" that might be mobilized against the detractor to achieve vindictive triumph).

Anyone wishing to deal effectively with physician executive leadership styles that reflect appeals to mastery, love, and freedom must find a balance between defending against, resisting, or changing the leadership style on the one hand and not making the executive too anxious and resistant to change on the other hand (which would have the effect of creating a greater reliance on the appeal). Low-key discussions in the physician executive's office are less threatening than public confrontations. Offering approval when merited is appropriate. Offering special readings on leadership and management styles might promote self-reflection and also permit meaningful discussions of the executive's leadership style. If respect from the physician executive can be developed, it might be possible to influence his or her leadership style at key moments. For example, when decisions are consistently made without involving others (autocratically), the suggestion that task groups be formed to gather more information might be accepted and thereby avoid a decision being made that is then rammed into implementation by the leader. In contrast, a leader that avoids making decisions can be encouraged to make decisions by providing him or her thoughtful analyses that explain the advantages and disadvantages of each alternative and a recommendation. Yet another avenue of pursuit is for the administrator involved to model adaptive managerial behavior.

And last, and perhaps of greatest importance, it is important that the administrator not become caught up in the compelling interpersonal dynamic that the defensive leadership styles create. There will always be the tendency on the part of the administrator who is the focus of the behavior to feel angry when nitpicked by a perfectionist, to fight back against vindictive attacks, to respond positively to nice but manipulative treatment, to take care of and perhaps rescue the helpless physician leader, and to accept all the responsibility if abandoned by the leader. Understanding these responses to the leadership tendencies permits administrators to avoid becoming overly anxious and emotional and permits an intentional response.

In sum, there are no easy answers to the problems some physician executive leadership styles create. Dealing effectively with them requires insight into their underlying causes and the courage to take the risks to counteract the behavioral patterns without, in turn, becoming manipulative or self-destructive. The next section examines the contribution more traditional organizational attributes can make to dealing with physicians and physician executives. Formal organizational elements provide important structure that helps to limit anxiety by providing clear direction and process. The remainder of this chapter is devoted to exploring the interactions of formal structure and personality.

Medical Group Governance

Medical groups are often filled with more than their share of difficult decisions and interpersonal conflicts. The lack of clear decision-making guidelines can encourage dysfunctional leadership styles and promote the formation of special interest groups that pressure medical group members, leaders, and administrators into courses of action not necessarily in the best interest of the group. As a result, careful consideration should be given to developing bylaws that direct medical group operations and decision making. There are a number of specific attributes that a well-conceived and comprehensive set of bylaws should include. It should be acknowledged that the importance of and formality of these considerations will co-vary with size and complexity. A small group of physicians who work well together and are in constant contact with each other might need little formal structure. In contrast, a large multispecialty group with a number of sites and many employees can benefit from codifying them.

A Mission Statement

The bylaws should start with a description of the group's purpose. What does the group commit itself to accomplishing? The statement should describe the group's purpose in overall terms and not become too specific or involved in the setting of goals and objectives. For example, a mission statement might read as follows:

> The Clinic has as its mission to serve the health care needs of the public. Services offered will emphasize primary general care but will also provide select subspecialty care. The Clinic will provide services in a manner consistent with high levels of patient convenience, accessibility, and availability. Services will be rendered in a professional manner that provides patients with dignity. The Clinic will be service oriented. Staff will provide prompt and courteous patient processing, including the sensitive handling of patient appointments, waiting time, registration, fee billing and collection, and ancillary services.

Membership in the Group

The bylaws should describe the criteria for membership in the group. This criteria might designate special types of membership such as partner, practicing member, or stockholder. There should be no doubt about how membership is determined.

Rules of Order

Robert's Rules of Order are often relied on; however, they may be modified or unique rules of order developed. In the latter two cases, the rules should ensure that clear discussion and decision-making processes exist.

Meetings

The frequency of governance meetings should be set forth along with the means for notifying members of the time and location. Provisions for special meetings and notification should also be provided.

Committee Structure

Permanent committees and how members are to be selected should be described. The preferred work methods for committees should be set forth along with guidelines for liaison and reporting to the governing body. Work methods might, for example, include the development of specific roles for group members, informal communication with members of the governing body to keep them up to date, and the proper method for documenting funding needs. Guidelines might include specified periods for the preparation of formal reports, accounting for the expenditure of funds, and the means for dealing with problems that might arise when crossing organizational boundaries. A provision should also be made for the appointment of special committees. Small groups of less than ten members might not need to develop committees; however, larger groups should consider them, especially when subgroups and committees have already been informally created.

Records

Minutes of meetings and subcommittee meetings should be maintained. The transmission of minutes to members should be described. Medical group partnership and incorporation papers should be handled with care. Copies of the papers should be kept on file, and the originals should be placed in a safe deposit box. Care must be taken that the originals and all copies are kept up to date as changes are made. A copy should be available to clear up differences in recollections on what was said.

Clear and Coordinated Task Assignments

Committees are frequently developed based on both permanent and temporary needs. Regardless of the need, committees work best if they have a clearly defined task. A clear statement of task is not easy to develop. Thought needs to be given to such things as the definition of the problem, the history of the situation, the impact of the situation on the group, and the expected outcomes. Clear task definitions help coordinate committees with each other and with the work of committees in the past.

Clear Authorization

Power and *authority* are two words that never fail to attract one's attention. Professionals are especially aware of the issues they raise. Committees often take on a life of their own, especially if they have vigorous leadership. Committees and leaders of committees might find considerable latitude in defining their authority, which can lead to the intimidation of other group members or departments, turf battles, confusion, and demoralizing conflict. It is important to define a committee's authority or empowerment before it starts to work. The authorization should include the consideration of who the committee may interact with inside of and outside of the group, what it can request and how, the extent it can obligate the group to a course of action, and the relationship of the committee's authority to any other potentially conflicting sources of authority in the group. On the other hand, committees need to be sufficiently authorized to carry out their work. Preoccupation with withholding or delimiting power and authority can result in unrewarding activity and conflict. When a committee's leader and membership are blocked from carrying out their work by a lack of proper authorization, negative feelings result. The proper balance of authorization is critical for successful committee performance.

Accountability

Committees must be held accountable by the group's leadership. A clear reporting structure should be specified. The structure should include both the timing of reports and the format. Accountability also requires the development of measures for performance. It should be agreed early on exactly what a committee is to accomplish and when. Accountability can be extended to the work processes of the committee as well. Some guidelines for work processes might be provided to ensure smooth operation of the committee. Some examples of these guidelines are the protocol for notifying the group's leadership of actions being taken to carry out work; the protocol for relating to other committees, members, and sections of the group; the measures for reporting progress; and the methods for recruiting members.

Goals and Objectives

The establishment of goals and objectives can have a stabilizing influence as they form a basis for directing decision making. Decisions should support the achievement of objectives and the fulfillment of the goals, all of which fulfill the mission statement. Additionally, establishing measurable objectives permits medical group members to determine the degree of success they and their leaders are achieving.

Policies and Procedures

The development of formal and often written policies and procedures that govern routine decision-making and administrative processes makes organizational life more predictable and less subject to the arbitrary whims of a few. Policies and procedures should not be unduly restrictive, although it is appropriate to expect them to exercise reasonable constraints over some administrative areas. The presence of agreed-to policies and procedures also informs staff who are often obliged to administer them and new staff who must learn what is expected.

The Intersection of Governance and Leadership

Thus far the formal attributes of governance have been discussed. The development of formal governance processes must also take into consideration the following aspects of organizational life.

Proactive versus Reactive Leadership

Another way to look at leadership in the health care environment is whether it is proactive or reactive. Proactive leadership is forward looking and action oriented. Developing a strategic planning strategy and then carrying it out is regarded as proactive. Actively searching out problems and correcting them is proactive. By comparison, reactive management results in crisis management. Problems that could have been foreseen and avoided are not. When things get bad enough, action is taken. Proactive leadership involves taking risks and requires energy to be expended. Reactive leadership involves little risk taking (nothing is ventured). However, reactive leadership creates another form of risk, the risk of not operating the group at its highest level of performance (nothing is gained). Care should be taken to understand when proactive and reactive leadership are appropriate.

Followership versus Acceptance

Leaders need followers. Followers have responsibilities for supporting leaders. Support does not involve unquestioning loyalty or submission to autocratic, totalitarian leadership. The group and its leadership benefit from the critical thinking of its members. Leaders, their styles, and their decisions should always be questioned. This recommendation should not be interpreted as authorizing nonconforming behavior. However, followers must not give up all their authority to their leaders. As colleagues, physicians often delegate authority and do not subsequently question those they authorize. As a result, physician leaders can come to perceive themselves as omnipotent. Members of medical groups who act as followers must be certain to assume their full responsibilities as followers.

Effectiveness

Effectiveness depends, in part, on the style of leadership offered and accepted. Autocratic leadership, for example, produces quick results while not necessarily fully considering all aspects of the problem or incorporating all the information and strengths the group possesses. Democratic leadership can result in good feelings on the part of members but produce slow and nondirected outcomes. Leaders who (1) vary their behavior based on the needs of the group, (2) provide clear direction, and (3) act to resolve conflict and uncertainty can produce outcomes that fit within preestablished time boundaries while maximizing the advantages of groups. Effectiveness, therefore, is not so easily determined. Groups that create conflict and bad feelings within the group or outside the group are usually considered to be ineffectively lead.

Conclusion

Understanding what makes medical groups tick is critical to working effectively with their owners and operators—the physicians. This chapter has highlighted the importance of appreciating some of the underlying psychodynamics of physician executive leadership styles and discussed some of the aspects of formal organization that might help to balance any negative effects of these leadership styles.

Notes

1. T. A. Jensen, "Physician Executive Leadership," *Medical Group Management* 33, no. 5 (September/October 1986): 20–26, 30.
2. M. Diamond and S. Allcorn, "Psychological Barriers to Personal Responsibility," *Organizational Dynamics* 12, no. 4 (Spring 1984): 66–77.
3. K. Horney, *Neurosis and Human Growth* (New York: Norton, 1950).

8

ASSESSING MEDICAL GROUP MANAGEMENT AND BUSINESS SYSTEMS

When the decision is made to network, hospital administrators must appreciate that medical groups can become complex organizations as more physicians, staff, and services are added. Hospital administrators must avoid the temptation of believing that how a hospital is operated readily generalizes to the operation of a medical group. Medical groups develop many unique management processes and strategies as a result of their collegial governance and leadership styles.

This chapter provides checklists to help hospital administrators assess medical group management and business systems. The content of the chapter is, in part, organized around a patient's encounter with a medical group. This approach emphasizes an operations point of view. The chapter begins by evaluating appointment, scheduling, and reception systems and continues by assessing internal marketing, which includes the experience of patients who pass through service areas, staffing, the administration of ancillary service areas, and medical record administration. Also covered in this chapter are assessing purchasing and inventory management, billing, accounting, productivity measurement, and managed care contracts.

Before continuing, the reader is reminded that the checklists are not exhaustive. They include fundamental questions that should set off additional spontaneous observations and questions on the part of those conducting the assessment. The first checklist relates to a patient's initial contact with a medical group.

Appointments and Scheduling

Patients expect to receive prompt, courteous attention when they call for appointments. Personnel who handle the phones and make appointments must appreciate the critical importance of this contact as it forms the basis for much of the patient's attitude and can turn the patient away. These personnel must be trained to have good telephone and people skills and to be able to use the medical group's appointment and scheduling systems effectively.

There are manual and electronic patient scheduling systems that range from elementary systems using an appointment book to completely computerized systems that have integrated appointment and scheduling functions. The type of system used depends on the size and needs of a group, the financial resources available to it, and the satisfaction of the physicians and staff with the current system.

A second aspect of appointment and scheduling systems is whether they are centralized or decentralized. Physicians in a large medical group might share the services of secretaries who schedule appointments manually. This method is usually preferred by physicians who do not want to "submit to the tyranny" of a centrally managed system. On the other hand, a manual, decentralized system can reduce the overall operating flexibility of the group and produce less operating and management information and information that has questionable accuracy. Modern appointment and scheduling software, when placed on a local area computing network, can provide the balance needed between local use and the power of a centralized system.

Assessment Checklist

- Is the system's performance reviewed annually?
- Has the system evolved as the practice has grown?
- Has computerization been considered in the case of a manual system?
- How quickly are patients scheduled?
- What are some of the complaints staff have?
- How effectively does the system handle complex appointments that require coordinating a visit with two or more physicians and ancillary services?
- Does the system generate useful operating and management reports?
- How difficult is the system to learn to use? Is adequate training and supervision provided?
- What kinds of system errors are most common? How is information about errors compiled and reported?
- Does the system provide timely and accurate scheduling information to clinic personnel? Is the information handled efficiently and cost effectively?

For computerized systems:

- How fast is the system? Do operators have to wait more than a second or a few seconds for the data entry screens to change?
- How user friendly is the system? Are screens laid out intelligently? Are they filled to the limit with data entry prompts and do they look overwhelming for the user?
- What kinds of reports are generated? Is the system accessible to all users, or are parallel manual systems also used?
- What kinds of backup arrangements are there for data files and system failure?

It should also be appreciated that the linkage of an appointment scheduling system to the collection of preregistration data is also an important convenience to patients and a time saver for the group.

Reception and Registration

Patient encounters with a group must be positive to further encourage a sense of professionalism, trust, and confidence on the part of the patient who, by his or her acknowledging a need for health care services, might be anxious. Receptionists must be pleasant, helpful, and know how to collect registration information, check preregistration, or confirm existing information quickly. Patient's should not have to stand in lines, and privacy should be provided. A number of aspects of reception and registration should be checked.

Assessment Checklist

- For patients who are preregistered, is the information accurate and has insurance coverage been verified?
- Have managed care patients been provided preauthorizations if necessary?
- Is complimentary "About Your Visit" information available to patients?
- Are all questions promptly and properly answered?
- Are personnel courteous and well trained in the use of the registration system?
- Are there complaints from billers about missing, inaccurate, and incomplete information? How much mail is returned due to misinformation collected during registration?

Internal Marketing Issues

Internal marketing is defined as all efforts that ensure patients have positive interactions with the medical group, including visits, communications, and billing. Internal marketing involves the management of the physical and service environment so that patients experience their treatment as favorable. All aspects of the facilities, grounds, and parking should be evaluated. Shortcomings in these areas can translate into much additional investment to bring the group's setting up to speed.

Assessment Checklist

There are many aspects of internal marketing. Some of the more important areas to check are the following:

Waiting room

- Is there enough seating? Is it comfortable? Is it conveniently located? Is it visually appealing? Is it comfortable? Is it maintained and clean?
- Is special seating provided for patients who are disabled?
- Is the waiting area crowded?
- Is lighting adequate?
- Is it appropriate to provide television?
- Are sufficient and interesting reading materials provided that are consistent with the interests of the patient population served? Are reading materials provided for all age groups, ethnic groups, and men and women? Are plastic holders used? How are magazines stored when not in use?
- Are toys provided for children?
- Does waiting room and service area decor contribute to the patient's sense of the medical group being of high quality and well managed? Are colors, floor treatments, wallpaper, or wood trim dated? Are art work and other accent items in good taste and changed occasionally? Is it clean?

Rest rooms

- Are rest rooms modern, well maintained and supplied, and clean? Do they contribute to the patients' comfort and ease of mind and to the perception of the medical group as maintaining a facility that patients will want to visit again?
- Are private rest rooms available for patients who must provide specimens?

• Are rest rooms located conveniently near waiting areas?

• If common rest rooms are provided as part of the building, are they properly maintained?

Parking

• Is convenient parking provided that minimizes walking distance?

• Does the group provide parking validation or passes when, for example, patients pay before leaving?

• Is adequate handicap parking available?

• Are parking areas well thought out for access, passage through, maneuvering for parking, and exit back onto the street?

• Do they have good lighting, and are they clearly marked?

• If a security guard is needed, are security personnel uniformed, pleasant, and helpful?

Climate control

• Are temperature and humidity controlled throughout the group's facilities? In particular how is the heating and cooling load handled throughout the day as the sun changes position?

• Are blinds used to best advantage to adjust not only for the sun's heat but also for glare?

• Is the system designed properly for controlling the temperature of each room?

• Are patients who have had to put on gowns monitored to see if they become too cold?

• Are portable electric heaters used in the winter? Are fans used to best advantage in the summer?

• How are smoking areas, if provided, ventilated?

Patients' experience of their visit

• Are floors, walls, windows, furniture, rest rooms, clinical spaces, administrative areas, grounds, and parking lots kept clean and in good repair?

• Are infectious and hazardous wastes properly disposed of and safeguarded from patients and children?

• Is it clear how patients request assistance after they enter a clinic room?

• Are signs easy to read and understand and provided where needed?

- Do gowns and robes meet patients' needs for privacy and warmth? Any savings in cost on purchasing cheap gowns and robes can be lost many times over in the negative experiences they might afford patients.
- How are patient valuables safeguarded if they must disrobe?

Flow of patients through the clinic

- How long does it take to process them through registration?
- How is basic physical information collected and when?
- How long do they wait in clinic rooms before being seen?
- Are all patients treated in a manner consistent with good judgment?
- How long do they wait for ancillary services, and where do they wait?
- How are they treated at laboratories, therapy, and radiology?
- How easy is it for patients to find their way about in the facility?

Personnel Administration

Good personnel administration is important for groups of all sizes. Personnel administration includes an assortment of functions: position classifications and specifications, wage and salary administration, interviewing and placement, orientation and training, and the development of policies and procedures regarding such things as attendance, absence, promotion, and progressive discipline. Managing these areas requires time and adequate information. However, professional personnel administration has a positive effect on staff members and is appreciated by physicians.

Assessment Checklist

There are many aspects of personnel administration that should be reviewed.

Analysis of staffing levels

- Does the medical group have the right number of and type of staff?
- Are staff maldistributed? It might be necessary to perform work load analyses to make a determination.

Hiring

- Have staff been hired who are related to some of the physicians? Are there "untouchable" staff? Medical groups that hire staff without a manager usually have unresolved staffing and performance problems that need attention.

- Are staff over- or underqualified for their positions?
- How have physicians and staff been recruited and selected?
- Have viable pools of candidates for open positions been developed before selection?
- Have temporary employees from agencies been used to fill open positions?
- How has interviewing been conducted?
- How thoroughly have references and credentials been checked? The possibility of hiring a health care professional with false credentials, licensing, and work experience exists.

Training

- Are staff cross-trained?
- Have staff been provided adequate training? Are top management supportive of training?

Supervision

- Is there an organization chart? Are reporting arrangements for staff clear, or have staff made up their own rules about who reports to whom?
- How have supervision and evaluation been handled?
- Are supervisors educated in the proper methods of supervision? Has training been provided that helps them carry out their responsibilities?
- Have formal evaluations of personal attributes and skills been conducted and linked to raises and promotions?
- Has corrective action been taken to deal with continuing performance problems? Have progressive disciplinary actions been taken?
- What provision has been made to cover the absence of key employees?
- Is the staff loyal to the group and their work?

Compensation

- Are staff over- or underpaid relative to each other and relative to position titles?
- Are employees paid competitively? Does the medical group know what the customary pay ranges for the various types of positions in their medical group are?

Personnel administration policies

- Does the group have written personnel policies and procedures? Is it clear how employees are to report their time at work, how they are to report absences, and how much vacation and sick leave they accrue?
- Are adequate records being maintained on employees?
- Has the group collected exit interview information from departing employees? Turnover has a real cost in terms of reduced operating efficiency, training, and waste.

Health Care and Ancillary Services Rendered

There are many facets to the delivery of health care in a medical group. A large multispecialty group might have developed many types of testing and therapeutic services that help to spread their overhead. However, the larger the group, the more likely it is to be experienced as a complex, hard-to-understand, impersonal business staffed with many employees. Many variables need to be carefully controlled to ensure patients have a positive experience.

Assessment Checklist

- How convenient and user friendly are the initial taking of weight and blood pressure and other vital pre–physician visit information?
- Are patients checked on frequently while they are waiting to see their physician? In particular, if they are uncomfortable or in pain, is some effort made to make them feel better while they are waiting?
- Are services that are rendered by staff (such as the taking of an EKG) done professionally? Are the procedures explained to the patient? Are supplies available to patients to clean themselves up afterward?
- What is the average waiting time to see the physician?
- Do physicians take the time to explain their findings and recommendations to patients? Do they do more than merely ask if there are any questions (patients do not often know enough to ask questions or might well be intimidated by the physician)?
- When tests and other diagnostic services are ordered for the visit, are patients provided guidance on how to locate the services and what to do when they get there?
- Are the service areas well organized? Are patients received courteously and informed about what to expect? Are local waiting areas adequate (see

waiting room checklist above)? Is the physical well-being of patients who must wait more than a few minutes attended to?

- Are personnel who render the services well trained? Are they friendly and service oriented?

- When it is time for patients to return to the clinic room, are they escorted if they are feeling ill or confused?

Medical Record Administration and Billing Documentation

Completing medical records, as many hospital administrators are well aware, is often not a high priority for physicians and nurses. Getting records completed can be time consuming and require persistence and diplomacy on the part of medical group staff. However, completing medical records on a timely basis is to everyone's advantage. Health care professionals will find it easier to complete records when they can recall what occurred. Fee billing personnel can bill more quickly and without corrections, and medical records personnel will not find themselves involved in extensive tracking of incomplete records. And lastly, physicians will find a complete record should a patient return for follow-up care.

Assessment Checklist

- Are all services rendered documented in the medical record? Physicians should provide signed and dated notes of daily visits, consultations, and orders. Medicare, Medicaid, other payers, and patients expect to be billed only for services rendered. Medical groups that do not consistently develop documentation to substantiate their billings can expect to have complaints from staff and patients and negative audit findings.

- Are procedures performed on patients (at bedside, in hospital laboratories, or in the office) documented in the medical record and signed and dated?

- Are dictated notes transcribed as quickly as possible, reviewed, signed, and placed immediately into the medical record?

- Are nursing services likewise documented in the medical record?

- Are records of drug administration carefully maintained?

- Do other health care providers such as physical, radiologic, and respiratory therapists document their services with a written, dated, and signed note in the medical record?

- Are the results of radiologic examinations and pathology laboratory and clinical laboratory tests dated, signed, and routed to the medical record for immediate incorporation?
- Do the medical records reflect the services and supplies consumed in the delivery of patient care (for the same reasons as mentioned above)? Although medical records will not necessarily document each service or supply item used, the record of care should be consistent with fee-for-service and supply billings.
- Does a lack of complete, accurate, and timely medical record documentation frustrate billing and collection efforts as patients depart? Incomplete records result in missed billing opportunities and confusion on the part of the patient, who might realize billing is erratic or inconsistent from one visit to the next.
- Are avoidable patient care risks being incurred for lack of documentation? Incomplete medical records create unnecessary delays and risks for patients. Misfiled or missing test results detract from patient care delivery.
- Can costly dual record keeping between the hospital and the medical group be avoided? Medical groups usually maintain their own records of outpatient visits whereas hospitals maintain a second record regarding admissions and other services. This creates complexity when both records are needed to care for the patient. Medical records or copies of medical records might have to be transferred back and forth between a group and a hospital. In some instances physicians might insist records be copied, creating two complete medical records and the attendant problems of maintaining them. Problems such as these can make electronic records a time- and expense-saving opportunity.
- Is medical record completion being monitored? Are medical records being monitored on an ongoing basis by staff and periodically audited using a random sample? Are nurses and those responsible for filing medical records routinely screening records for completion after patient visits?
- Do fee-billing personnel find the medical records adequately documented and complete?
- Are there written medical record policies and procedures? The following are typical policies and procedures:
  1. A definition of what constitutes chart completion
  2. A specification of time frames for completing medical records
  3. A specification of how documentation should be assembled in the medical record

4. A specification of forms that are to be used in the medical record

5. A specification of the nature of the filing system for medical records

6. A specification of monitoring of record completion and reporting

• How adequate is the medical record filing system?

• Are there filing backlogs?

Purchasing and Inventory Management

Purchasing and inventory systems should facilitate the timely acquisition of the correct items at the least cost and achieve delivery where and when desired. Additionally, records of requests, orders, approvals, the receipt of merchandise or equipment, and payment should be maintained as an audit trail and for future reference.

Assessment Checklist

• How are supply inventories monitored? Are reorder points part of the system? How often are physical inventories taken?

• Are there too many supplies on hand? Are there remote storage areas and associated costs?

• Is there waste and spoilage?

• Are purchase requisitions used to provide exact information on what is to be purchased and its likely costs?

• Are purchases that involve large sums of money approved by the governing body? Are justifications provided that outline likely costs and revenues to be earned? Are such things as return on investment and payback calculated?

• Are bids usually requested from vendors for the purchase of expensive equipment and for large volume purchases of consumable supplies?

• Are written purchase orders used? Do the orders specify exactly what is being ordered, the amount, the cost, the location for delivery, the billing address, and a purchase order reference number?

• Are bills of lading used to check in the merchandise received?

• When the manufacturer's invoice is received, is it matched to the record of what was received? Is the record of what was received, the invoice, and the check presented to the administrator for signature?

• How are the invoice and record of what was received filed?

- If a computerized purchasing system is used, how adequate is it? Is it interfaced with an accounting system? Computerization will facilitate administrative research (ad hoc inquiry). Many records must be maintained on paper regardless of the sophistication of a computerized purchasing system. Orders, invoices, bills of lading, notices of receipt, vouchers, and checks all require paper, paper that must be related together and filed.

- What kinds of reports, analyses, and management information are developed from the details of individual transactions that are compiled and recompiled into summaries, reports, and information?

- Are reports, analyses, and management information accurate and representative? Reports might omit information that is useful in learning more about the purchasing system. Analyses might distort information by making improper comparisons or plotting trends that cannot be compared one to the other. The question is, do the reports and information tell the reader enough about what is going on to completely understand the performance of the purchasing system?

- What internal controls are in use? Purchasing systems are vulnerable to being manipulated for personal advantage. There are steps that can be taken to avoid the loss of control of purchasing systems. They include the division of duties, enforced vacations, cross-training, and central receiving.

- Are economical lot sizes being ordered that maximize discounts without creating storage and spoilage problems?

- Are rent or lease purchase decisions carefully explored? How many leases currently exist?

Professional Fee Billing

Professional fee billing is the life blood of a medical group. There are many important aspects to an effective charge capture, coding, and billing service. Hospital administrators must appreciate that professional fee billing is more complex than DRG-based hospital billing.

Assessment Checklist

- How do physicians report their inpatient and outpatient fees to billing staff? Does it ensure accurate and timely communication? Is it a user friendly process?

- How are diagnostic codes reported? Is the physician provided adequate information and a user friendly system?

- Are outpatients provided a complete and accurate superbill?
- How are authorizations from prepaid plans acquired? Are charge opportunities routinely lost?
- Does the group make any effort to routinely screen medical records for billing documentation?
- Does the group handle its billing and fee setting in a manner consistent with its legal organization?
- How trained are billing staff? Is a modern computerized billing system used? How well managed is it? Aged accounts receivable and collection experience should be reviewed.
- How does the group handle overdue accounts? Are several collection agencies used?
- Are there problems with insurance submissions?
- What is the history of the group's payer mix?
- Do billing staff report any chronic problems?

Accounting and Fiscal Administration

Medical groups can generate substantial cash flows that must be effectively managed. Annual average medical group operating expenses are around $150,000, and there are often complex salary and incentive arrangements for the physicians. Hospital administrators must take the time to learn about a medical group's accounting and fiscal administration.

- Are accounting and financial management handled by medical group staff or by a contractor? If handled internally, are the staff competent, and are sufficient internal controls in evidence? If handled externally, who in the group has been designated as liaison, and is the person performing the needed oversight functions? What kinds of monthly operating and financial reports are being generated?
- Are certified financial statements and tax returns available for review?
- Does the group have a debt structure, and if so, how cost effective and well managed is it?
- How are investments, if any, managed? How are surplus cash and reserves invested?
- Has the group negotiated low-cost bank services?
- Has the group developed a process of carefully monitoring retirement program costs? Are all liabilities funded?

Evaluating Productivity: Productivity Measures

Medical groups should have a program to measure productivity. There are several compelling reasons for productivity measurement. The group should have the ability to objectively compare physician productivity in terms of patients seen, procedures performed, billings, and income generated. In larger groups objective accountability is essential for meaningful discussions of physician performance and compensation. Similarly the group should be able to objectively compare the performance of staff, technicians, and ancillary health care professionals. This is essential to meaningful discussion of matters such as efficiency, discipline, compensation, and promotion.

The group should be able to assess the adequacy of equipment. A lack of information on operating efficiency can make it difficult to make informed decisions regarding changing equipment or purchasing additional equipment.

Additionally, a productivity measurement program serves to heighten the awareness of employees and physicians about their responsibility to meet established standards of excellence and productivity. And last, historical productivity data permits retrospective analysis of factors contributing to current operating problems and the evaluation of changes.

Any activity carried out by members and employees of the group should be considered a potential data element. However, care must be taken to narrow down the data elements to only those essential for determining productivity, and every effort should be made to collect the data as part of daily routines. Thoughtfully designed forms and software can facilitate the collection and processing of the data at a minimum cost in staff time. There are a number of questions that can be asked regarding the collection and use of performance data.

Assessment Checklist

- Is performance data shared with employees as a means of their assessing their own performance? Most employees are interested in doing a good job, and meaningful feedback is one of the keys to their adjusting their behavior to accomplish better work.
- Is performance data analyzed for trends?
- Is performance data compared to industrial standards and to other medical groups that might wish to share performance information?
- Are trend analyses performed on the following aspects of a group's practice?

1. Patient visits by day, by physician
2. Time in the clinic per physician
3. Time in governance and administrative meetings for physicians and staff
4. Number of laboratory tests performed by hour
- Are data collected on the following aspects of the practice?
  1. Number of patients seen per hour, per physician
  2. Number of patients turned away without an appointment
  3. The number of no-shows
  4. The number of incomplete or unacceptable laboratory tests
  5. Total patient time at the clinic
  6. Professional fee billings per physician broken down by procedure
  7. Collection experience by patient category, by physician, by third party payer, by service rendered
  8. Amount of professional courtesy granted, indigent patient care, and bad debts
  9. Productivity per hour, per day of ancillary services

Evaluating Managed Care Contracting

Medical groups can, as a result of not thoroughly analyzing the effects of managed care contracting or managing the effects on an ongoing basis, find that they have compromised their financial stability. Hospital administrators must take the time to review all managed care contracts for advisability; to understand how they are or are not being managed; to evaluate their contribution to operating margins; to appreciate their effect on patient referrals to the group; and last, to understand how the contracts relate to the hospital.

Assessment Checklist

- Are there complete, current, and accurate records for all managed care contracts?
- Are there executed agreements, and did an attorney review them?
- Are group-prepared analyses available?
- Has the group developed a management information data-collection and -processing system that monitors managed care contract performance?

- What kinds of routine day-to-day problems are encountered in dealing with the staff of managed care organizations, their paper work, their authorization systems, and their reimbursement methodology?
- What are the interactions between managed care contracts and between the contracts and market share?

Evaluating the Medical Group Manager

Hospital administrators must take care in evaluating the performance of a preexisting medical group manager. These managers can range from secretaries who have worked their way up to educated and qualified medical group managers who are the equal of hospital administrators. The evaluation process can be approached indirectly from a number of perspectives.

Assessment Checklist

- How does the manager conduct himself or herself at meetings with the hospital administrator?
- Does the manager prepare thoughtful reports and analyses?
- Are there sufficient business systems to generate management information?
- What use has been made of computers in managing the group?
- What types of credentials and experience does the manager have?
- What do some of the opinion leaders among the physicians and staff of the group think of the manager?
- Does the manager participate in local and national medical group management organizations?
- In general, how well run is the medical group's clinics and other enterprises?

Conclusion

Medical groups are complex businesses that deserve careful review by hospital administrators before launching into a formal affiliation with them. Many medical groups are operated by less than fully qualified administrators and, as a result, might have developed many chronic fiscal and operating problems that will require the investment of considerable attention and often negotiation to resolve.

9

LINKING HOSPITALS AND MEDICAL GROUPS VIA MANAGEMENT SERVICE AGREEMENTS

Hospitals can bond medical groups to themselves by offering a variety of services that will improve their practice operations while reducing costs. Hospitals that wish to become involved in the management of medical groups without venturing into ownership will find practice management service agreements a way to make the linkage. Service agreements can range from providing discounted medical supplies and equipment to providing professional expertise for strategic planning, marketing, and advertising.

The development of management service agreements creates a win-win outcome for hospitals and medical groups. Hospitals can expect to absorb many of the incremental costs for offering these services within existing cost bases while generating new income from direct or indirect cost recovery. An example of direct cost recovery is billing a medical group for services rendered. An example of indirect cost recovery is a hospital achieving a greater economy of scale in laboratory and radiology service areas. More patients are seen. Incremental income is captured. Overhead is spread over a larger service base. Medical groups that contract for the service will benefit from reduced costs, improved operations, and less expenditure of physician time on administration.

It should be noted that practice management agreements provide a safe arm's length relationship for physicians relative to hospitals. Management agreements should offer no real threat to physicians who fear that their practice will be taken over by a hospital. The agreements also assure hospital administrators that they will not become excessively entangled in the dynamics of the leadership politics of the medical groups that they provide services to.

Practice management agreements offer hospital administrators a number of additional benefits.

- They provide a friendly foot in the door to medical groups, thus strengthening their bond with the hospital.
- They permit hospital administrators and staff to develop more rapport with physicians.
- They provide a means for hospital staff to gain a better understanding of what is involved in managing medical groups.
- Successful agreements can be expected to lead to additional opportunities to offer hospital services and perhaps provide a basis for greater collaboration and the development of joint ventures.

Hospital administrators can develop this new function in a variety of ways:

- First, existing staff can be reorganized and pressed into service to support group practices. Hospitals that operate more than one site might find the development of these services an ideal opportunity to consolidate staff to gain even larger economies of scale while making it easier to develop these new services. A position of coordinator of physician management services marketing should be considered to provide a focal point for physicians to interact with.
- Hospital administrators can hire personnel who have medical practice management experience to develop and deliver a wide range of services to medical groups. Many hospitals are creating these special in-house consultant staffs to develop these types of services.
- Hospital administrators who do not want to commit their own personnel to organizing and delivering these services might want to consider contracting with practice management consulting firms to organize or provide these services. These consultants provide expertise to deal with practice problems while providing physicians a neutral party to work with in improving their practice.

There are many possible management services hospitals can develop to offer to medical groups. The balance of this chapter describes some of the more important ones. However, before proceeding, three words of caution are in order.

Words of Caution

Hospitals are not often looked on as benign and might, in fact, be perceived as unfriendly by physicians. They are also not often looked on as being efficiently operated. To the extent physicians hold these beliefs, developing service agreements will be made more difficult. As a result, hospital administrators who endeavor to develop these services must be committed to providing high quality services or risk alienating the physicians, who will be quick to pick up on problems. A major problem can strain the relationship, and the bad news can be spread rapidly throughout the local physician community, which might well undermine further efforts to market the services. There can be no substitute for doing an outstanding job.

A second consideration is that nonprofit hospitals, in offering new products and services that are unrelated to their mission, can jeopardize their tax-exempt status if they are not careful. Profits gained from these activities might be taxable. Hospitals should be aware of this possibility when structuring and pricing the services.

Hospital administrators can avoid tax problems three ways. First, if the service is related to health care delivery, it may be considered a related activity and not subject to taxation. Laboratory and radiology services provided to practice patients is an example of this type of related service. Second, the services can be priced to break even, thereby creating no profit to tax while providing some cost benefit to the hospital by spreading hospital overhead over a larger cost base. The resale of office and medical supplies at cost plus handling is an example where this strategy might work. And last, the problem can be avoided by not charging for the services. Services offered by professional administrators already employed by the hospital who can absorb additional work into existing work schedules can provide the service at little additional cost, thereby making it possible to offer it without charge.

The third caution is that hospital administrators should be careful to avoid violating safe harbor regulations and other related laws in making these types of agreements (see Chapter 6).

Purchasing Agreements

The easiest agreement to develop might be the purchasing agreement. These agreements permit medical groups to tap into a hospital's purchasing power and membership in, for example, purchasing consortia. Medical groups benefit from buying office supplies, instruments, and equipment at discounted rates. Hospitals that pass along some of the discounts that they receive create savings for medical groups while providing the hospital additional income.

The basic agreement can be enhanced by several additional offerings. A hospital might wish to go one step further and provide a wholesaler service where, for a small fee, common supplies are warehoused and delivered on demand to medical groups. This arrangement might be particularly practical if physicians maintain their offices on the hospital's campus.

A second enhancement lies in inventory administration, where inventory control, reorder points, quality control and economic lot size considerations are applied by specialized hospital staff to further improve the cost effectiveness of medical group management of inventories and purchasing. In addition, physicians can be kept apprised of the latest developments through an information service and seminars. This type of service can be particularly valuable when it comes to equipment purchases.

Purchasing equipment can be one of the most troublesome and unrewarding activities medical group administrators have to deal with. Complex equipment with many features, hard-to-calculate costs and benefits, hard-to-understand service agreements, and hard-to-assess vendor performance considerations can require a major commitment of physician time with the probable outcome that the decision made will still be less informed than that made by a hospital's staff that specializes in equipment needs assessment and purchasing. The purchasing department of a hospital combined with staff from such areas as business and information services, laboratories, radiology, surgical, and rehabilitation can help guide medical groups to wise equipment purchases especially suited to their practices. Additionally, hospital staff can help to install and debug new equipment, smooth operating procedures, and provide staff training to help medical groups to take advantage of their purchases.

Laboratory and Radiology Services

Laboratory and radiology services are costly and complex to offer. Frequent changes in technology, high front-end costs, space needs, environmental protection, and increasing regulation make owning or leasing laboratory and radiology equipment a time-consuming and costly enterprise that requires ongoing administrative attention to ensure that profitability is maintained. These considerations can make contracting with hospitals for these high-technology services an attractive option for physicians. The problems associated with purchasing and operating the equipment and safely disposing of wastes are shifted to a hospital that has sufficient capital and staff to deal with vendors and to operate the equipment in a safe, regulator-approved manner.

This option is made more attractive if the hospital constantly improves the professionalism and convenience with which the services are offered. These improvements, when combined with efforts to locate medical group offices nearby, make the service attractive for physicians and patients. Hospitals offering these services can further encourage their use by providing free patient transportation and specimen pickup and rapid turnaround of test results. Hospital administrators are also encouraged in this direction for economic reasons as economies of scale are gained by optimizing throughput involving expensive equipment. In sum, hospitals are usually better prepared to operate these services and can provide patients and physicians a valuable service that physicians can either contract for and continue to bill patients or simply direct their patients to for use.

Space Leasing

Many hospitals have empty and underutilized space that can be converted to generate income. A productive use of excess space is to rent it to medical groups at reasonable rates for their practices. In fact, many hospitals are building office space as part of their strategy to compete for admitting physicians. Modern, well-run, and contiguous physician office space is something physicians appreciate. The development of office buildings is leading to the development of large medical center campuses that include many kinds of services. Physicians and patients are attracted to comprehensive, modern facilities that offer many amenities such as convenient, covered, close, free, and safe parking; clean modern facilities and furniture; outstanding food service; and easy-to-access health care services.

Physicians might, in addition to finding it convenient, be encouraged to rent hospital space for more pragmatic reasons. While there are tax advantages to owning a building, there are also many disadvantages such as arranging financing, developing building plans, and operating and maintaining a building. Leasing is also no panacea. Physicians who lease space in buildings they do not control often encounter frustrating problems such as maintaining and controlling mechanical systems, the maintenance and replacement of carpeting and furniture in common areas, unpredictable security and maintenance, and poor parking. They might also have no control over who rents space in the building, which can lead to too much competition or the introduction of other businesses that are not compatible with the practice of medicine. A last consideration is that a practice might be asked to leave when their lease runs out, creating a disruptive and costly move. Many physicians see hospital-owned and -controlled space, while not magically solving all these problems, as providing them with a landlord who has a vested interest in keeping them happy.

Business and Information Systems

Medical groups and practices have many of the same business and information needs as hospitals. Hospitals can provide medical groups computer terminals and staff support that is made all the more easy by having practices located nearby. This approach, it can be pointed out, provides medical groups access to sophisticated technology, powerful hardware, state-of-the-art software, and trained business and information systems professionals. It also provides them with the opportunity to access computerized patient information, laboratory results, and electronic medical records without leaving their offices.

For example, the handling of accounting and payroll requires the preparation of checks, the recording of disbursements, the encumbrance of orders, and the complex calculation of employee taxes and benefits. Another example is patient scheduling, registration, and billing. Professional fee billing has gradually grown to the point where it is important to have professionally trained managers to handle it. Dealing with third parties and handling claims submissions, applications for payments, and collections efforts requires a constant level of attention to avoid the risk of lost income. The question that must be asked of physicians is why they should duplicate the resources of hospitals when hospitals can provide physicians business and information services with a higher level of expertise and likely at a lower overall cost. Why should medical groups make major investments in computers, software, and personnel when they can contract for these services? Should physicians be interested in these services, there are several levels of integration that can be considered. There are less integrated approaches where information can be batched and delivered to hospital personnel for data entry and processing. A second, more integrated approach is to develop computerized interfaces between hospital systems and medical groups systems to, for example, handle scheduling and registration.

Regardless of the approach used, it is always important to understand that physicians are inherently suspicious of possible lapses in confidentiality and security, losses of control of their information, lack of responsiveness to problems, time-consuming computer downtime, and slow screen responses, and they will always worry about paying for the hard-to-evaluate costs of these services. Hospital administrators must be prepared to persist in marketing these helpful but, at times, hard-to-understand services.

Human Resources and Benefits Administration

Human resources and benefits administration is yet another area that medical groups and hospitals must deal with and which hospitals are much better equipped to handle. Personnel and benefits administration can become complex and costly areas that, if not well managed, can result in avoidable costs; wasted time and effort; and unnecessary employee turnover, grievances, and law suits. This complexity, if physicians appreciate it, should encourage them to accept help if someone that they perceive can professionally handle their needs extends it.

Hospital human resources management staff can assist medical practices in many areas:

- The recruitment and screening of talented administrative and health care delivery staff, including arrangements for candidate travel and accommodations, interviewing, sightseeing, receptions, and house hunting
- Wage and salary administration, career tracking, and staff development
- The development of detailed position descriptions and job specifications and a scheme for classifying the positions relative to each other and organization charts
- The development of progressive discipline policies and personnel evaluation processes
- Supervisor training and continuing medical education opportunities for employees, including record keeping
- The development of policies and procedures for all aspects of a practice's personnel administration

A lengthy list of possible areas of assistance can educate physicians about what they should know and bring the sobering realization that they are not informed. The development of a proposal can be substantially aided by the use of a ready-reference audit checklist that documents missing elements in the management of a medical group's personnel.

Practice Marketing

The 1990s will be a decade of ever increasing competitive pressures on hospitals to keep admissions up and increase the utilization of ambulatory services. During the 1980s hospitals pioneered direct patient marketing methods. Typical examples have been the marketing of urgent care centers, specialized mental health units, and birthing units. However, the growing realization that these efforts do not match the influence physician gatekeepers have has, once again, attracted the attention of hospital marketeers to achieving better connectedness to physicians.

The 1990s will see the new trends in joint hospital-physician marketing and the providing of marketing services to medical groups to help them support their marketing efforts to gain market share.

Joint Marketing Opportunities

Hospitals and medical groups can find many health care services and programs that they have a common stake in developing. There are many examples where more effective marketing by half of this equation benefits the
other half. It is then perfectly natural to look at how to combine forces to
gain marketing synergy. Some examples of joint marketing opportunities are

- sports medicine programs that involve hospital radiology, surgery,
  and rehabilitation services;
- cancer treatment services that span a broad range of physician services such as pain management and in-office chemotherapy and
  hospital services such as bone marrow transplant, nuclear radiology,
  and surgery; and
- kidney disease treatment programs that involve the supervision of
  patients by physicians, physician supervision of chronic dialysis clinics, and, for hospitals, acute dialysis treatment and kidney transplant
  programs.

Increasing public awareness of the sources of these types of services or,
perhaps more accurately, product lines is a critical factor in increasing the
size of the marketing pie and increasing the size of one's piece of the
pie. In sum, joint marketing opportunities can greatly expand competitive
effectiveness and must be explored.

Medical Group Marketing Services

During the 1990s hospitals will provide medical groups sophisticated marketing services to help their admitting staff to build a larger share of the
market. These services might include

- the design and implementation of advertising campaigns;
- the creation of promotional opportunities and materials such as highly
  visible shopping mall blood-pressure screening, brochures, and patient newsletters;
- the development of special events such as open houses and health
  fairs;
- the development of a public relations program that takes advantage
  of free publicity opportunities; and
- market research and assessment including test marketing required
  to produce helpful insights that avoid costly clinic and product-line
  expansion mistakes.

Strategic Planning

Strategic planning has become a necessity for medical groups if they are to maintain or increase their market share. Unfortunately, strategic planning is not often a high priority for physicians, who might also hesitate to involve hospital staff in this important and confidential aspect of their practice. Strategic planning services are, nonetheless, an area of high potential intercompatibility, and they can eventually become a necessity if physicians and hospitals are to develop plans that avoid duplication and optimize the use of marketing resources. For example, hospitals must be careful to avoid developing product lines that will conflict with and eventually anger their admitting physicians. Similarly, physicians should be careful to avoid planning a new venture that will overburden available hospital services. Another example involves hospitals that, having developed strategic plans, have also acquired a great deal of data and information about the local marketplace that can be used to facilitate medical group planning efforts. Closely related, hospitals that have long-range planning will also have developed information systems that track, on an ongoing basis, all kinds of trends such as diagnoses, referring physician admitting patterns, and payer mix patterns.

The development of planning and information systems is an expensive, difficult, and time-consuming activity that need not be duplicated by medical groups if hospitals are willing to share their information with medical groups. Medical groups that are prepared to join with the hospital in planning will enjoy the advantage of accessing all this information that will, when combined with hospital planning expertise, permit rapid, thorough, and effective planning that is integrated with the plans of the hospital.

An area related to strategic planning is the analysis of long-term financial planning for medical groups. Hospital financial staff can provide highly useful services in the areas of cash management, budgeting, internal control, cash flow analysis, variance reporting, cost projections, and financial analyses.

In sum, integrated strategic planning for hospitals and medical groups will become an essential exercise for medical groups in the 1990s to achieve the competitive advantage planning has to offer.

Management Assistance

Physicians are finding that running a medical practice is a complex and difficult task. Many are turning to outsiders for help. Physicians are now often looking to hospital administrators for help in managing their practices. Many hospitals are responding by providing temporary assistance and, in some instances, permanent management support for medical groups (Chapters 10 and 11). The key question for hospitals in offering management services is whether the confidence of the physicians can be earned. Physicians will be concerned that they are selling out their interests to the hospital, which will then pursue its own interests to their detriment. Physicians might also remember unpleasant confrontations with hospital administrators whom they no longer like or trust. In sum, marketing management services to medical groups requires patience, and offering temporary support services is a good way to open up these linkages.

There are many areas hospital administrators can help physicians with. Temporary assistance is often sought to overcome a broad range of pressing operating problems, to buffer ongoing administrative problems for those groups that do not employ a practice manager, to span a period of time when turnover necessitates recruiting a new manager, and to assist practice managers in highly specialized administrative areas such as computing or human resources administration. The following are some specific kinds of services that can be offered:

1. Management engineers and internal auditors can review and improve clinic operating procedures using their systems analysis skills. These skills, it may be pointed out to physicians, include mapping patient services for delays and inconveniences, the assessment of paper flow and accounting procedures via flow charting, and perhaps most important, review of the professional fee billing systems for charge capture, throughput control, employee compliance, collection efforts, and operating costs. There are many areas these professionals can scrutinize for inefficiencies and opportunity costs that can be pointed out to physicians.

2. Hospital business office staff can help their counterparts in physician offices to improve their methods for managing payroll, accounting, accounts receivable, and inventory. A good example of where this kind of collaborative relationship can be helpful is in the exchange of patient registration information for professional fee billing. Many times physicians provide inpatient services and do not gather registration and insurance information that will permit their bill to be submitted for payment. Clinic billing personnel are then stuck with the time consuming problem of contacting the hospital to obtain the needed information either from the patient's medical record or from the hospital's computerized registration information system. How easily this is done depends on how good the working relationship is between the two staffs and whether modern information

management and electronic communications systems are used to share information. Hospital staff can guide medical groups to computerized access to the hospital's registration information.

3. In the medical arena, hospital nursing, laboratory, radiology, utilization review, and quality assurance staff can advise and train physicians and clinic staff in their areas of expertise. For example, nurses and technicians can provide continuing education to help clinic staff keep their skill levels current. Another example is in the areas of managed care and Medicare, where hospital experts on utilization review and quality assurance can advise physicians on how to meet requirements on a timely, convenient, cost effective basis while avoiding unnecessary duplication with the hospital. Hospital staff and physician collaboration is also essential in the areas of cost containment and reduced length of stay to optimize hospital profitability and DRG reimbursement.

These and many other areas form the basis for developing an administrative services program for medical groups. Given that providing these services might involve a considerable time commitment, hospital administrators might wish to charge out these costs to physicians, who might be more than willing to pay a fair price for good service.

Patient Convenience Services

Hospitals can find other services to help physicians improve their patient care. For example, small medical groups might not be able to afford staffing at times outside normal practice hours and therefore not be able to deal effectively with the emergent health care needs of their patients. Hospitals that provide courtesy rooms for physicians to use to see their patients outside of their usual office hours benefit all concerned. Physicians see their patients without worrying about extra staffing costs, and hospitals benefit by reducing the volume of subacute care delivered in their often overworked emergency departments. At the same time, a service such as this has a marketing advantage in that the hospital is, it is hoped, found to be a nice place to visit.

Conclusion

There are a number of reasons why hospitals should develop medical practice management services. First, physicians will be appreciative. For example, they should find hospital assistance is quicker, more informed about local

conditions, and cheaper than hiring consultants. They might also find contracting for ongoing services more cost effective than hiring additional staff
and purchasing or leasing additional clinic equipment and space. Second,
admitting physicians will become much more attached to their hospital,
securing for the hospital a stable base of admitting physicians. Successfully
competing for admitting physicians will be a key element to the long-
term financial viability of hospitals in the 1990s. Third, hospitals that offer
outstanding management services can expect to turn them into direct and
indirect income-generating opportunities.

However, this win-win approach is not without pitfalls for hospitals.
In particular, physicians might be suspicious of a hospital offering the same
service to their competitors. Fears might develop about how to safeguard
proprietary information when a hospital deals with a number of practices.
For those physicians who view the hospital administrator as the enemy, the
offering of these services to physicians might look like an attempt to control
the physicians. As a result, regardless of whether the service is good or not,
they might not allow the hospital anywhere near their practices. And finally,
hospitals interested in providing these services must learn to work with
physicians and must learn the business of practice management to do well.
The services must be outstanding to be seen as beneficial to physicians.
Poorly designed or delivered services reflect badly on hospitals and have
an effect opposite the one intended because ongoing relationships with the
hospitals key resource—their admitting physicians—are threatened. Hospital
administrators must be committed to spending the time and money to plan
this type of venture and make sure they have the personnel to deliver an
outstanding product.

The following case example highlights much of the content of this
chapter. The case is based on a real example. The names of the organizations
have been changed.

Case 9.1
Midwest Hospital Corporation and
Northland OB/GYN, P.A.

Northland OB/GYN, P.A., a seven-physician, multiple-office obstetrics and
gynecology medical group located in a large city, has developed management
problems. The physician who founded the group 20 years ago has begun
to phase out his practice and give up his leadership role. He expects his
colleagues to assume additional administrative responsibilities and to locate
a new leader in their ranks, all this during a time of growth that is creating
new operating problems. However, no one is willing to step forward to

accept the formal leadership role, and as a result, the physicians are creating an executive committee charged with dealing with the growing number of unresolved operating problems.

Foremost among the problems is staffing. The group suffers from high physician turnover due, in large part, to dissatisfaction with ineffective leadership and administrative problem solving. This turnover and difficulties in recruitment have resulted in too few physicians to adequately staff existing practice sites and a complete inability to develop new services. Employee morale is also suffering from the leadership vacuum. The group's nurse manager, for example, reported feeling handcuffed and unable to deal with many of the problems because of the lack of decision making.

The deteriorating situation has attracted the attention of several of the newer physicians, who have been working hard to develop high quality services. They feel that they have to find a way to turn the group around, and they are assuming proactive leadership roles in the executive committee. They are also quickly discovering that they were not familiar with management and operations, have no experience in directing and supervising a manager and staff, possess little knowledge of how to plan for the growth of their practice, and, as a result, realize they prefer to practice medicine rather than manage their practice.

The Northland physicians are major admitters to two of Midwest Hospital Corporation's area hospitals. Their practice generates an impressive volume of procedures and deliveries for the hospitals. The physicians have heard through the grapevine that Midwest is making all kinds of deals with doctors in the area, either buying out their practices or supplying them with capital to keep them solvent. As a result, the executive committee has decided to contact Midwest for help in dealing with their pressing problems.

During their first meeting with Midwest's representatives, the physicians learn the hospital corporation is most interested in helping them out. The representatives propose a management agreement whereby Midwest assumes responsibility for providing day-to-day management of the practice. The physicians immediately agree.

To start, Midwest proposes that a local practice management consultant be retained to evaluate the practice and make recommendations about what to do to get the group back on track. This is agreed to, and a consultant is hired to review the practice's staffing, operations, morale, management, and governance. The consultant's recommendations are presented to the executive committee by the staff accountant Midwest assigned to manage the practice. Most of the recommendations are accepted, and the staff accountant is charged with implementing them.

In addition to getting operations straightened out, the agreement also calls for Midwest to help the group with physician recruitment, provide technical assistance with developing a computer system, work with the group to develop a strategic plan to deal with future growth, and provide a line of credit to help stave off cash flow problems related to the buyout of the retiring physician's equity in the practice.

Analysis

This case illustrates a typical hospital-physician service agreement approach. Northland is a group practice experiencing a difficult leadership transition where the founding physician is turning the practice over to group members who are unwilling to take the reigns from their leader of many years and who are also unprepared to assume management responsibilities. As a result, chaos is developing, and the physicians look for help from an interested third party, in this case, from Midwest, whom they had heard might help out.

Midwest accepted the invitation for a number of reasons:

1. Midwest is paid for services provided by existing staff who found the time to work with the group.

2. Had the group failed, the two Midwest hospitals involved would have experienced a major loss of admissions.

3. The invitation also provided Midwest an opportunity not just to maintain the group but also to expand it, further increasing the group's market share and by extension the market share of the Midwest hospitals.

4. The invitation provided the two hospitals involved an opportunity to add additional services that the physicians wanted to add but had not.

5. A successful relationship was expected to encourage other area physicians to approach Midwest for help, thereby further strengthening Midwest's competitive position.

The physicians of Northland contracted with Midwest for good reasons:

1. They needed help managing their practice and financial assistance with their cash flow.

2. They felt comfortable working with Midwest personnel, whom they had, in some instances, known for years and trusted. At the same time, they avoided having to deal with their fears and ignorance and the uncertainty of hiring a practice manager whom they might then feel at the mercy of.

3. They also saw advantages in developing a long-term affiliation with Midwest. The group had no plans to change sites or admitting

hospitals. They had also developed a good reputation in the area, which supplied them with many patients. Developing a better working relationship with Midwest made good sense for the long run.

Longitudinal Problems

Longitudinal problems arise even from the best of agreements. As time passed, the staff accountant assigned to the group did not have the time to attend to all the problems that arose. Additionally, this individual was not familiar with operating a practice and, despite good accounting skills, was often ineffective. As a result, the executive committee developed many complaints about their administrative support.

The computerization of the practice also encountered delays and difficulties. The hospital's computer staff were asked to select and implement a new computer system for the group; however, they quickly learned that they were not dealing with a hospital system. A practice, they discovered, had different appointment scheduling, patient billing, and medical information management needs. And even though they knew how to select hardware, they were unfamiliar with clinic practice software applications and had to struggle to make adequate choices. They also partially undermined the implementation of the system by not having sufficient time to spend with the practice to effect a smooth implementation.

And last, as the group became more secure with the financial backing of Midwest, their requests for plans, space, equipment, programs, and staff increased. Midwest administrators began to feel that the physicians were treating them like a bank. At the same time emboldened Midwest managers decided to exert more control over the decision-making processes of the group, which substantially increased tensions with the physicians. Open hostilities occasionally broke out, and hard-to-resolve conflict developed. The honeymoon was over. However, because a long-term agreement had been signed, both parties gradually realized they had to try to keep the tensions to a minimum by working together more effectively while permitting the practice and the Midwest hospitals each to optimize their unique interests relative to each other and without anyone feeling they were being abused or taken advantage of.

Summary

The case illustrates the good news–bad news aspects of developing management agreements with medical groups. To tap their positive aspects, hospital administrators must diligently avoid the negative aspects.

10

MEDICAL GROUP AND HOSPITAL JOINT VENTURES AND SHARED OWNERSHIP OF MEDICAL GROUPS BY HOSPITALS

Shared-service arrangements and contracting for management services are some of the least involved ways that physicians and hospitals can network. These options enable each party the advantage of working together without having to give up ownership and autonomy. The next level of integration in the spectrum of hospital-physician networking is the joint development of a health care delivery entity or the shared ownership of a medical group. These two approaches tie the hospital and physician participants together as partners. This chapter examines issues physicians and hospitals face in forming joint ventures or in sharing ownership of a medical practice. It focuses on how to deal with structure, governance, management, operations, financing, and participant behavior. To begin, joint ventures that create a third, new entity are discussed. However, before jumping into the development of a joint venture, the parties involved should make sure that they are interested in working together.

Before Pursuing a Joint Venture

Parties to a venture should share a common reason for being involved. Each party should need something that the other party has in order to achieve its objective. These days, physicians are often looking for business assistance, capital, or partnership security from a hospital. Hospitals are usually seeking new sources of revenue, and they need physicians to generate hospital business in the form of admissions and the development of competitive new products. There are, therefore, financial and nonfinancial reasons for pursuing a joint venture. The following are some of the more common financial reasons:

- Increasing the market shares of the respective partners by creating new marketing opportunities. A hospital and a group of cardiologists might, for example, create a joint heart center that increases the recognition of the hospital and the members of the medical group in the prevention and treatment of heart disease.

- Gaining a source of capital. Chapter 2 discussed the difficulty physicians have in accumulating funds for capital expenditures.

- Obtaining a more competitive position with local third party payers, especially HMOs and PPOs. The collective strength of a hospital and one or more medical groups can force a plan to renegotiate its contracts.

- Diversifying the types of products a hospital offers. Payers are tiring of paying for hospital inpatient services. Increasing the stake that hospitals have in the outpatient market is becoming a necessity.

- Sharing financial risk with another player. Managed care capitation arrangements assume providers are willing to work together to manage care. Joint ventures encourage hospitals and physicians to work together to manage accompanying costs.

- Avoiding costly duplication and taking advantage of economies of scale. Hospitals and medical groups compete with one another in a market that does not welcome costly duplication and encourages economies of scale. Joint ventures permit direct accomplishment of these important tasks.

There are also nonfinancial reasons that hospitals and physicians might wish to form a joint venture:

- Gaining long-term practice and institutional security. A medical group that ventures with a hospital can establish a highly defensible market position, thereby providing security from competitive pressure.

- Achieving institutional, medical group, and personal goals. An urban, religious hospital might have as one of its goals providing care to the poor and underserved. The creation of a community clinic that is staffed by volunteers from a medical group fulfills this mission as well as perhaps goals of the medical group and some of the personal goals of the physician involved.

- Enhancing the public image of the hospital and physician group. Ventures, while making money, also provide new and improved services to the community.

- Utilizing the nonfinancial resources of one partner that are not available to the other partner. New ventures require the planning and marketing of new treatment modalities to get them off the ground. Hospitals have employees who can develop the needed planing and marketing while the physicians must develop the skills needed to offer the new service.

More than likely, one or many of these reasons might contribute to the decision of a hospital and medical group to form a joint venture. However, no matter what the reasons are, the key to success lies in the ability of the partners to act like partners. Physicians and hospital administrators come from different personal and professional orientations. Physicians, who value autonomy, must decide if they will be comfortable in giving up some of their decision-making authority. In turn, hospital administrators must be patient with the often slow, deliberate decision-making processes of physicians who often find business dealings stressful and something that is avoided. Both parties must also have a clear understanding of their goals for participating in the venture, and they must also appreciate the goals of their partner. Both parties should feel that their respective goals can be met and that one party does not gain disproportionate advantage.

Several additional considerations are that the partners must feel that they gain synergy from the common objectives and that they must strive for mutual trust and respect. The latter outcome can be particularly difficult to achieve between physicians and hospital administrators. Lack of good faith in the past can lead to a struggle for control of the venture between the hospital and the medical group as each acts unilaterally to protect their respective interests from the other. This lose-lose dynamic will eventually reduce if not completely cripple the utility of the venture. Both parties must appreciate that their joint product is primarily the services provided by physicians. The success of a freestanding ambulatory surgery center, for example, lies in its use by surgeons and not its association with a hospital. Hospital administrators must accept this fact and try to keep the hospital's real value to the venture in perspective. They must particularly accept that the primary role of the hospital might be that of the financial-management backer of the venture.

Developing Hospital-Physician Joint Ventures

Joint ventures in health care delivery can take many forms and include many things. They can encompass facility construction (medical office buildings), medical equipment (imaging machines), product research and development (biomedical), or the operation of a clinic or a medical practice. Hospital-physician joint ventures are today relatively unique and somewhat controversial. As nonphysician parties (hospitals, pharmaceutical and medical device companies, and medical services management firms) become involved in patient care, they are attracting considerable scrutiny from lawmakers. Chapter 6 discussed the legal implications and concerns regarding these relationships. They want to prevent abusive referrals to such ventures by persons who benefit financially. This issue is the litmus test that potential venturers must pass and must be kept in mind when developing hospital-physician relationships.

Initiating a Joint Venture

Potential new ventures must first be assessed for feasibility. In particular it must be determined that the market will support the new or expanded service. Also to be determined is who should join the partnership. There are two important membership issues. First, physicians in the right specialty must be found. A cancer center, for example, can be staffed by oncologists or in a multidisciplinary format that includes radiologists and surgeons. It must also be appreciated that interspecialty politics, payer reimbursement, and personal conflicts might ultimately serve to decide which partners the hospital has to work with. Also to be examined is the business nature of the medical groups being considered. A conservative group might be unwilling to look at alternative health care delivery programs. Physicians who are not willing to take risks and try new ways to deliver care are not going to be good partners when the hospital is considering innovative new programs.

The second issue for a hospital in planning joint venture participation is whom to include or exclude. A decision not to invite a particular physician, type of physician, or group to participate in a venture can ruin its chances for success. Exclusions must be talked through with all stakeholders to build as much consensus as possible among the members of medical groups and within the physician community. For example, in the cancer center example, a medical group might have a well-known oncologist who, after many years of practice, wants to retire. The hospital's administration also knows that the physician, while maintaining good practice standards, has not kept up with the most progressive treatment modalities. However, the group and physician community are expecting that this physician will head the new cancer center.

The hospital wants the cancer center to be state of the art and would like to hire a leading oncologist from a nearby medical school to head the program. As a result, many members of the group and some physicians in the community are upset with the intended direction and feel that the physician deserves a chance at the role as a result of his or her loyalty to the hospital and community. At this point the hospital administrator has a tough problem on his or her hands. The image of the center can be enhanced only at the risk of alienating many admitting and potentially referring physicians. Compromise might regrettably be in order.

Typically, the hospital administrator can and will use the medical affairs director or physician services director to help make these decisions and sell them to medical groups, medical staff, and the physician community. The hospital administrator should make sure that key players are contacted and briefed early on in the planning process. Discussions in the doctor's lounge can often make or break a new venture.

Once the partners are identified and approached about a possible joint venture, they must determine what each party wants from the venture as well as what they can bring to it to make it successful. Several important questions need to be answered. (1) What does each partner bring to the venture? (2) What is each partner's objective in participating? (3) Why does that objective need each partner involved? (4) What is each party willing to give up in the venture? (5) Are the objectives of all partners compatible?

Participants, particularly physicians, might not want go through the exercise of answering these questions. There are two reasons why this often happens. First, the exercise requires the parties to show their cards up front, which implies trusting one another in what amounts to a rather frank discussion of mutual goals and objectives. Trust might be sorely lacking. Second, physicians tend to look at these ventures like investments. If they are successful, great. If they are not successful, they will get out. This cut-and-run approach is often be discerned by hospital administrators and creates reservations on their part, especially if the hospital is fronting millions of dollars. In addition, the physicians might look at the venture as being more important to the hospital than to their group unless it clearly has a major influence on the medical group's practice.

In sum, a great deal of attention needs to be paid to accessing the feasibility of a joint venture. The politics between hospitals and physician groups can greatly influence the outcome if the participants are not careful to discuss all aspects of the venture. The partners must be patient in feeling each other out and in gaining an appreciation of their respective positions and objectives.

The Key Elements of a Joint Venture

The key elements of a successful joint venture are the proper handling of the development of corporate structure, governance, and management, including budgeting, billing, finance, and the operation of the new service.

Corporate structure. Joint ventures typically involve the creation of a new entity that is jointly owned by two or more partners. The entity is more than likely a for-profit corporation or partnership. Partnerships can be arranged to have all members be equal partners, or there can be one general partner and several limited partners. The venture is sometimes nonprofit or a foundation whose proceeds support educational or research efforts.

The work involved in creating a new legal entity can be extensive. The development of a large venture might require the partners to form an executive committee to deal with the many administrative matters and decisions that need to be made. Doing the actual leg work in setting up the corporation is usually best left to attorneys and accountants. The partners might also find it helpful to retain a management consulting firm to help them through the steps of setting up the venture. Hospital administrators must keep in mind throughout the process that the key physician decision makers might be busy seeing patients and have difficulty making meetings, thereby making the process painstakingly slow for the hospital.

There are many time-consuming and complex corporate issues that need to be decided. Some of the more common ones are, (1) Will the new entity be hiring its own employees? (2) Under what entity will services be billed? (3) Who will manage the day-to-day operations? (4) Where will the entity be located? (5) How will investment capital get into the corporation? and (6) What equipment will be needed for the entity? These are all important questions involving how the venture will be run.

Governance. The most critical element of the new venture undoubtedly involves its governance. Problems can arise when one of the partners wishes to assume or actually assumes a role of leadership that is greater than that of the other partners. A typical situation involves a hospital administrator who, after creating a venture, grows impatient with its slow development and takes a much more proactive leadership role in the interest of expediency. The physicians involved will likely see this move as an attempt to take over the venture and use the physicians as pawns in the hospital's marketing battle with a competitor. A problem such as this can be mediated by the development of a governing board (a steering committee or formal board of directors) that provides a formal means to avoid dominance by one party. The bylaws of the venture can also be written to include, if necessary, unanimous votes on important decisions, to further ensure balance.

Medical groups should look at how representation on the venture's board fits into the governance structure of their respective organizations. Each group should decide whether it is better to have their highest leadership or the people directly involved with the venture sit on the venture's board. A second critical aspect of this question is whether the representatives are empowered to commit their respective organization's resources to meet venture needs. Board members most often have to bring issues back to their leadership for approval. For example, hospital administrators often assign an assistant administrator to sit on a joint venture board and limit his or her ability to commit the hospital's resources. The assistant administrator essentially attends these meetings as the representative of the administrator. However, care must be taken that this form of limited empowerment does not lessen the dedication of the partners to working with one another to achieve their common and individual goals. In particular, care must be taken that those who sit on the governing board have comparable empowerment from their respective organizations.

Business planning. One of the biggest tasks facing a new board is the creation of a business plan. This plan, beyond putting the concept of the venture into operation, must create a credible management structure, define each partner's role in the operation of the venture, develop the financing needed to get the venture underway, provide for a legal review to ensure that the plan stays within legal boundaries, and establish a time line for each of these actions to be completed.

Board members need to remember that even the best laid plans are subject to change. Flexibility in decision making must be maintained so as not to ruin a venture over simple issues such as what the stationary should look like.

Budget, billing, and finance. The joint venture should have a budget to guide its financial needs and to permit the evaluation of its performance. The budget should include both development costs and a projection for the first three years of operation. There are several good reasons why joint venture partners must develop and maintain budgets. Budgets provide the participants with a guide for how much of a financial commitment they must be willing to make in the project. A project can sound exciting in discussion but take on a totally different tone when financial reality is tested. It is wise to be sure that the physicians involved understand the financial implications of the project unless the hospital wants to provide the only deep pocket for the venture. In particular, since many physician corporations do not accumulate large sums of capital, it is important that they understand the financial reality of their planned venture obligation. All too often, tragedy strikes hospital-physician joint ventures when the physicians get in over their financial comfort level. The relationship can then become strained, and the venture might collapse, forcing the hospital to buy out the disenchanted physicians.

A second good reason for budgeting is that it provides the partners with an assessment of whether the venture is meeting its financial objectives. The commitment of each partner to the project might have been based on a pro forma budget projection that showed the venture either breaking even or making a certain level of profit. If the financial reports show less than this, the partners might want to reexamine their commitment to the project or change it to get it back on track financially.

The specifics of the financial arrangement of the venture vary by the type of venture created. The biggest factor involved in professional services ventures is whether the entity takes in its own revenue or bills through the hospital, the medical group, or both. An example of the latter situation is a wound care clinic where physicians and hospital staff team up to care for patients with wound healing problems. The venture operates like a physician's office; however, the physicians take their billings back to their offices, and the hospital does the same with facility charges. The entity itself does not charge patients for services and therefore has no ongoing financial support to pay for operations. As a result, the partners have to devise an equitable financial arrangement to pay for the cost of its operation.

Management and operations. Unless the venture is going to be run by either existing hospital staff or the physician's clinic staff, the venture needs employees. The amount and type of staffing depends on how large and freestanding the entity is. Some ventures require hiring a large clinic staff (receptionists, nurses, business office staff, and managers). In contrast, some ventures, such as jointly owned satellite medical offices, require relatively few incremental employees. For example, an arrangement where the venture purchases or leases space that the physicians use as part-time satellite offices might be staffed, in part, by the physicians who bring with them staff that they need to deliver care. In this case, the venture's only permanent staff would be receptionists to schedule appointments and answer patient questions and perhaps radiologists and laboratory staff as needed. These venture staff are economical to hire since their costs are spread among all the physicians using the facility.

The size and sophistication of the venture also determines whether a full-time manager should be hired. Hospital staff can successfully manage some ventures as part of their day-to-day responsibilities. For example, functions such as accounting, personnel recruitment, marketing, and purchasing, as mentioned in Chapter 9, can be handled through hospital departments and coordinated with the venture by an assigned administrator. However, it is critical that it be clear that this administrator reports to the governing board or to an executive committee of the board to once again ensure balance in the working relationship.

Larger, more sophisticated ventures need a dedicated administrator to ensure that business plans are followed and that desired levels of success are achieved. Several factors might influence the decision of a board to hire a full-time administrator:

- The politics of the creation of the entity might dictate that a neutral person be hired. If the position is assigned to a member of the hospital's management staff, the physicians might feel that this person's allegiance is to the hospital. The hospital might feel the same if the person comes from the medical group. Having the venture entity employ an administrator who is subordinate to the board provides the needed sense of neutrality.

- The complexity of the entity might demand that a full-time administrator with skills in clinic management, physician billing, health care finance, personnel management, marketing, and data processing be hired.

- The specialty nature of the services provided may require a person who is familiar with the product line. An example of this is a home health service staffed by home health aides and nurses. The board might want to hire a nurse with experience in delivering home health services as its administrator to ensure product quality. Management problems with a service company such as this more often occur in the delivery of the service than in the administration of the business.

A person that the hospital administrator does not want to ignore in the venture development process is the medical group's administrator. There are two reasons for this:

- The physicians have developed a working relationship with and trust in their group's administrator. They work with this person daily, and they want to hear his or her ideas and comments on how the venture should be structured and how it will affect the practice's operations. Hospital administrators should pay attention to any sensitivity that develops on the part of the practice administrator as arrangements for the venture progress. For example, the venture might involve considerable integration of the medical group's functions, so much so that if a new manager is hired for the venture, the existing manager might feel he or she has been displaced.

- The venture involves services in the specialty area of the physician. The group's administrator will be knowledgeable about the potential problems of offering a service in the group's areas of expertise. Billing issues, such as what to charge, how to code the services, and how to establish relationships with third party payers, are one example of where an experienced administrator can be very helpful. If the venture board decides to use management support services (i.e., billing, payroll, accounting) that the physician's practice can provide, the administrator will have an ongoing administrative relationship with the operations of the new entity.

In sum, hospital-physician joint ventures are challenging to develop and challenging to maintain. Many of the challenges faced have been discussed. Many of these challenges apply equally well to the development of shared ownership arrangements.

Shared Ownership of Medical Practices

Hospital involvement in the ownership of medical groups is one of the fastest growing trends in the hospital industry. This activity has moved to the top of the hospital administrator's agenda as he or she deals with declining revenue. Hospital-physician joint ownership of medical groups has come about as physicians have invited hospitals to share in both the management and equity of their practices. These arrangements involve issues similar to joint ventures; however, they are different in one important way. The entity involved (the medical group) already exists and is totally owned by the physicians. This is critically important for hospital administrators to appreciate.

The importance of this issue is not necessarily financial or business related. It is primarily of psychological importance. The involvement of a hospital in a medical group is something new for physicians. Physicians might initially feel comfortable with the idea of sharing the business side of their practice with an outsider. However, as discussion continues, they might come to feel that they are compromising control over their practice. They might feel that the hospital is invading their group by getting involved with its finances and operations. Hospital administrators must appreciate these feelings and fears to be successful negotiators.

Developing Shared Ownership of a Medical Practice

Earlier chapters have suggested reasons why physicians might want to involve hospitals in their medical group. The following are some of the most common reasons:

- They might need capital to continue to grow and to meet the growing needs of their patients.
- They might need financial assistance to stave off cash flow problems, including bankruptcy.
- They might need management and technical support services.
- They might wish to be included in the hospital's provider network for long-term patient flow stability.
- They might want help in accommodating risk-sharing capitation contracts with HMOs.
- They might want to secure a funding source to guarantee that the physician's buyout will occur when he or she is ready to retire.

Hospital administrators are reminded that the items in this list are based on the development of a relationship between a medical group and a hospital in which the hospital's predominant role is that of banker. Hospital administrators must fully appreciate this view as they work with medical groups. Appreciating the other side's motivations and agenda is critical to developing a successful collaboration.

Organizational Structure

Many states prohibit outside interests from owning equity in a physician PC. As a result, the hospital administrator must develop a different legal-structural approach to networking via shared ownership. Typically, these approaches involve the creation of a separate entity to which the medical groups sells its "hard assets," such as clinic buildings, computers, medical equipment, clinic furnishings, and accounts receivable. The new entity, in purchasing these assets, provides the group the sought after capital. The essence of the arrangement is that the hospital is loaning the medical group money and is using the hard assets of the group as collateral (see Figure 10.1). This new entity can also choose to hire the medical group's employees and, in turn, contract them back to the group for management and support services. By adding this piece, the new entity gains considerable control over every aspect of the group's practice except its clinical activity. At the same time, the hospital's involvement enables it to facilitate the group's growth.

Governance

The creation of a new entity not only facilitates the flow of capital but also provides the partners with a new forum for joint decision making. Commonly, the boards of these entities include equal representation and require a consensus-building approach to decision making. The level of involvement by the hospital's board representatives varies depending on the status of the group's practice. Typically, the greater the problems, the more extensive the hospital administrator's involvement in decision making. In contrast, when the hospital is merely providing capital to help a well-managed, trouble-free group to expand, the hospital's representative might remain a silent partner, allowing the physicians to maintain control over their group. However, should a well-managed group experience some difficulties, the hospital administrator might want to closely monitor the group's progress in solving the problems to protect the hospital's investment. In this case a position on the board grants him or her the authority to directly participate in the group's management if necessary to ensure progress is being made. It is recommended that the hospital administrator discuss his or her desired level of involvement with representatives of the medical group during the negotiation process to avoid any unacceptable surprises.

The level of involvement of the hospital administrator also depends on whether he or she has long-term objectives for the relationship. If so, more involvement in the planning and direction of the group's activities

Figure 10.1   Shared Ownership Organization Structure

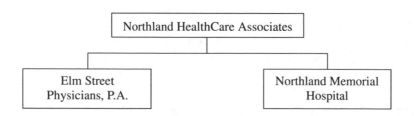

is indicated. However, if the intention is to provide a short-term fix to a problem, he or she might assume the role of a silent partner.

Board Size

The size of the board varies depending on the size of the group. A potentially sensitive issue that hospital administrators should be aware of is that, prior to the involvement of the hospital, all the physicians in a group might have participated in the group's decision-making process. Taking on a hospital partner requires the individual physicians to give up some of their direct participation and power to hospital representatives. As a result, the physicians might have trouble trusting the board to represent their interests.

Changing Patterns for Problem Solving

A group that takes on a hospital as a partner might also see the problem-solving behavior of its members change. Traditionally, physicians have felt free to represent their own interests in dealing with group problems. However, when a nonphysician partner enters the picture, the physicians often respect their new partner's position even when it is not consistent with their own. Hospital administrators must be sensitive to this point. The physicians will have run their business their way for many years. The presence of a hospital administrator at the decision-making table will be a new and strange experience for the physicians. As a result, the partners must develop a comfort level to work together. The hospital administrator should be up front with the group about the role he or she intends to play relative to financial and management issues. The administrator should also remember that he or she is on the group's turf. The hospital administrator must work to establish rapport with the physicians and show respect for their individualistic nature while demonstrating that his or her participation is for the betterment of the group's practice.

Financial Issues

One of the main reasons hospitals are invited to buy into physician practices is for the hospital's deep pocket. Regardless of whether the hospital's contribution is structured as a loan that physicians are expected to repay or as an investment in the group's hospital revenue-generating potential, the hospital owns a stake in the affairs of the practice. The financial involvement of the hospital should be discussed thoroughly with the physicians since it can raise many questions. Some of the common questions are these:

1. How long will the hospital be involved with the practice?
2. Will the physician's compensation package change?
3. Will the debt repayment arrangement be difficult for the cash flow of the practice to accommodate?
4. How will the financial obligation to the hospital affect physician's buyout arrangements?
5. Will the hospital's contribution provide enough working capital to improve the practice's situation or is it only enough to bail out the current situation? and
6. Will the infusion of dollars be once or ongoing?

Limiting Involvement

It is important that the arrangements and terms for the hospital's contribution be consistent with the circumstances. A wide-ranging involvement in a group is inappropriate if the practice needs only a short-term loan to handle a physician buyout. A group that is not able to come up with the dollars needed to fund the retirement of a senior physician and that received unfavorable bank terms might be forced to turn to the hospital for assistance. In this case, the group usually offers some of its assets as collateral, including a portion of future earnings to secure the loan. However, if the hospital administrator sees this as an opportunity to gain control over the group and thus proposes a much more involved and lengthy arrangement including a strategic planning process and a management contract, the physicians might well balk at this and walk away from the deal.

A struggle for control is a lose-lose situation. It is wiser for the administrator to go slowly in structuring arrangements with physicians. The goal of any arrangement should be to meet the needs of the situation to build trust. In the above case, the physicians were only looking for a loan and not a long-term relationship. Hospital administrators should view these opportunities as a way to demonstrate to the group that the hospital is willing to provide assistance. As a result, it is hoped that the physicians will feel that the hospital is a good partner and initiate or welcome discussions of new ways to explore their relationship. Patience is required to develop a strong and trusting relationship.

Hospital administrators must also appreciate that they need to be careful that agreements are not perceived as benefiting only certain members of a group. The buyout of senior partners is a good example. If handled poorly, the younger physicians can perceive this type of an arrangement as the senior doctors looking out for their own interests at the expense of the rest of the group. Consequently, the hospital administrator appears to support these older members to obtain what he or she wants. Once this occurs, restoring the trust of the remaining physicians can be expected to take a long time and much effort.

Accounting

The accounting mechanics for the joint ownership of a practice by a hospital can be complex. Typically, the process is as follows:

1. The hospital contributes cash to the entity to be used for development.
2. The physician's professional corporation sells assets to the new entity. The outcome of these two steps is that the hospital receives the physician's assets as collateral for the cash invested.
3. If the physicians desire to purchase back their assets, they must negotiate buyout terms with the hospital.
4. If the physicians want to have the hospital as a permanent partner, the assets can remain split between the two, and new purchases can be held in common.

The new entity also needs to be careful about how it bills patients for services. Physicians are required to bill for services under their own name. Payments made to the physicians are then signed over to the corporation for deposit. An exception is payments from Medicare and Medicaid. In their case the outside entity may not purchase these accounts receivables from physicians or receive payments made to the physicians. This exception requires the new entity to work out a method to deal with it.

Management

Dealing with the issue of management can be the most difficult problem the parties face. Like with joint ventures, both parties might have reasons for either using existing staff or recruiting new staff. The difference here, however, is that the management function manages the medical practice and not a new entity. If the practice does not currently have a manager and it is mutually agreed that one is needed, then the parties need to work out how they want to approach hiring. The options are (1) to recruit and hire a manager to run the practice who will work for the practice and report to the board of directors or (2) to contract with the hospital's clinic management company to lease management and staff to manage the practice.

There are advantages and disadvantages to these options. Hiring a manager requires the person to report to the shared governance of the group's board. As discussed with joint ventures, the main concern is that the administrator remain neutral in his or her allegiance. The manager cannot be viewed as being manipulated by the hospital to influence physician behavior in such areas as longer hours, more patients seen per hour, or seeing patients at different clinic sites. Should issues such as these arise, it is recommended that the administrator stay out of the middle of the debate or risk losing rapport with the side that loses in the decision-making process. It is important that the administration be allowed to concentrate on improving problem areas, and this task is best accomplished by avoiding a struggle between the physicians and the hospital over who controls what.

If the practice currently has an administrator, then the parties need to discuss their evaluation of his or her performance before deciding how to proceed. If the practice is having horrendous problems that are directly attributable to the administration of the practice, the decision seems clear cut. However, if the physicians are generally pleased with their manager and the hospital is not, a problem invariably develops. Hospital administrators must keep in mind during an encounter such as this that the physicians trust the administrator and might even be irrationally loyal to the person. As a result, change must be approached with exceptional care and ingenuity. An example of the ingenuity required might be convincing the physicians that it is wise to add one of their administrators to the milieu as a form of balance. The physicians might also be coaxed into accepting a consulting company to take a look at the situation or contracting with a management service organization. In all of these instances, the administrator is left in place (at least for the time being) without necessarily sacrificing opportunities to improve management. However, even these approaches can run into stiff resistance from the administrator, who can still win the day.

The second option above, while possessing economic and efficiency advantages, can be problematic as well. The main advantage is that the hospital might have an effective management structure that will allow the practice to plug into its many services (see Chapter 9). In this scenario, the new entity contracts with the hospital to provide the services desired. Here again, if the physicians are concerned about their management structure being under the control of the hospital administrator, then this model will not be accepted. If pursued, there is one primary issue that the hospital must address: quality. Physicians with experience in going this route often complain that the personnel and services provided are not geared toward medical practice management. They complain that the various services provided are tied too much into the hospital's structure and do not allow enough flexibility to meet the needs of their practices. In particular medical groups might experience frustrating limitations to hospital data management systems and personnel recruitment processes. Additionally, it is always risky to let hospital business office staff handle physician billings. Professional fee billing requires staff who have considerable experience in managing physician billing systems. Hospitals must deliver a good product that is orientated to medical practice to be seriously considered by physicians and medical groups.

Conclusion

In summary, joint ventures and shared ownership of medical groups offer hospital administrators a foot in the door in building a relationship with medical groups. The key to success for both parties is to be a good partner. It should also be kept in mind that, even though physicians have dealt with hospital administrators on hospital-related clinical matters, joining with a hospital as a partner in a separate business venture is a new experience. Physicians are invariably reluctant to give up the control of their practice to a hospital administrator with whom they have not always been on the best of terms. However, in a market in which purchasers are now expecting hospitals and physicians to work together to provide good quality care at a contained cost, these avoidance tendencies must be overcome.

Case 10.1
Metropolitan Sports Medicine Center

Lakeview Medical Center (all names are fictitious) had planned to become a regional tertiary care center for orthopedic and sports medicine. Spine care, foot and ankle surgery, and joint replacement clinics had been developed, and the next step was to add a sports medicine program to capture the local professional athlete market as well as that of the sports minded public.

A large orthopedic group, the Smyth & Jones Orthopedic Group, was also interested in developing a center of excellence in sports medicine. The group had orthopedists who served as team physicians for several of the local professional teams. The group's leaders learned of Lakeview's plans in the sports medicine arena. At about the same time the group's management determined that, because of the large investment involved, an area hospital's support would be needed.

Discussions between Lakeview and the Smyth & Jones Group eventually took place and led to the notion of developing a joint venture for the opening of the Metropolitan Sports Medicine Center (MSMC).

The MSMC board of directors was to comprise two hospital representatives and two physicians. The business plan called for the hospital to
provide ambulatory space and specially equipped orthopedic surgery suites
that would be exclusively committed to the center's use and, by extension,
to the group's physicians.

During the planning process the hospital administrator learned that
orthopedists from one other major orthopedic group felt that they were
being snubbed by the closed planning process. They expressed an interest
in participating in the joint venture as they feared Lakeview would create
a super group that would seriously damage their practice. The hospital
administrator appreciated their concerns and decided that it was politically
correct to open up discussions to include all area orthopedists. After months
of, at times, heated meetings, it became apparent that the Smyth & Jones
group and other area orthopedists were in direct competition with each other
and that they could not join together in the venture. In the end, the original
plans were followed.

When the center was finally opened, it was operated as a stand-alone
outpatient facility. The Smyth & Jones Group provided the patient information system and the physician billing and collection system. The hospital
provided reception, nursing, radiology, and additional staff as needed and
billed separately for ancillary services that it provided on site. It was also
expected but not obligatory that most major surgical cases would be admitted
to Lakeview.

The opening of the MSMC was followed shortly by the opening of a
second sports medicine clinic developed by the second orthopedic group. The
group's leaders, despite having been included in discussions, were angry that
Lakeview's management had shown favoritism. The leadership of the group
also feared that their big new competitor would hurt their practice. They
had decided that the only possible response was to open their own sports
medicine clinic. This was accomplished in a joint effort with a physical
therapy center located in a fast-growing, affluent suburb.

In addition, other orthopedic surgeons who practiced at Lakeview
began to experience a drop in their referrals because referred patients seemed
to be going to the now highly visible MSMC. They were also dissatisfied
with the operating rooms that were available to them, which were not as well
equipped and not always available at convenient times. As a result they began
to move their practices to other area hospitals that were more supportive.

Case Analysis

Lakeview's objective of developing an outstanding orthopedic and sports
medicine program was realized but at the expense of creating an aggressive

new competitor and alienating other orthopedists on its staff. Lakeview's management did not adequately appreciate the competitiveness of medical group practice. Siding with one group was eventually viewed as unfair and threatening. Losses of admissions from the alienated physicians, when combined with the activities of the new competitor, compromised Lakeview's success.

Hospital administrators should be careful about how they position themselves relative to medical groups. When there is more than one major specialty group represented on its staff and within its primary geographic market, care must be taken when considering opening a major new center or program based on only one group's exclusive participation. It might be wiser to expand participation in joint ventures to permit all groups and practitioners to participate equally.

Case 10.2
Midwest Hospital Corporation and Family Physicians of Deerfield, P.A.

Midwest Hospital Corporation (all names are fictitious) owns and operates several hospitals, including one in rural Deerfield. The Deerfield hospital had for years been struggling to maintain a positive bottom line as other area hospitals increased their competition for Deerfield patients. The hospital's survival hinged on maintaining the viability of a number of family medicine practices.

Deerfield was served by a handful of family practice physicians who, as a result of the deteriorating local economy, were having difficulty maintaining their practices. In particular, some of the younger family physicians had been lured back to Metropolis, where they could earn more. The remaining family practice physicians had been borrowing money from Midwest to keep their practices afloat. Their individual situations eventually led them to consider joining together to improve their finances by forming a family practice group.

The development of a group presented them with the following opportunities:

1. The physicians could reduce their costs by sharing services, including clinic space, staff, and business systems.
2. They could stabilize themselves financially by consolidating their individual loans from Midwest. The group could approach Midwest to permit them to transfer their individual debts to the new group practice using their accounts receivable as collateral.

3. Midwest could also be approached to provide the financial resources that were needed to deal with staffing and salary level problems that contributed to overwork and dysfunctional employee turnover.

4. Midwest could be asked to extend a major loan to the group to purchase a new computer to support a clinical information system and professional fee billing and collection.

5. Physician time spent on administration could be reduced. Together they could afford to hire a medical group manager.

6. Each practice had contracted with a local HMO, and they were all losing income to the plan. A new contract was needed that pooled their capitation and brought the Deerfield hospital into the risk-sharing arrangement.

7. Their group could approach physicians in nearby communities to join with them in developing a primary care network.

8. Merging their practices would allow them to deal with operating problems such as on-call coverage and managed care contracting.

The management of Midwest was receptive to the idea of helping the physicians develop Family Physicians of Deerfield, P.A. The development of a group would likely ensure the success of the Deerfield hospital. They agreed to provide the financial support requested but with some stipulations. First, Midwest's management asked that the group expand its size and add pediatrics and obstetrics. Midwest would assist in the recruitment of new physicians. Second, the Deerfield hospital would build a new clinic for the group on the hospital's campus. This would provide them with a convenient practice site. Third, Midwest agreed that they needed to recruit an administrator and that they had to invest in more staff and equipment.

The first stipulation initially bothered the group. They were concerned that becoming a multispecialty group would create factions within their group. The group liked the idea of a new clinic as long as the hospital was going to pay for it and provide them with a favorable lease. Hiring an administrator was fine, but they wanted the person to report only to them.

After much debate the physicians decided that they wanted Midwest's support but only as a banker to finance their development. They felt very strongly that they should maintain their independence and wanted to keep the hospital at arm's length in the development of their group practice and clinic. This was agreeable to Midwest but with the stipulation that, given the size of the loan, a management representative of the hospital participate in group business meetings and be consulted about major decisions.

New problems arose during the consolidation of the individual practices. The group began to realize that the practices of some of the partners
were not profitable and would have to be changed. The hospital provided an
interim administrator to support the group; however, the physicians seldom
had time to meet with her to address the many problems they were facing.
The group had also not anticipated all the financial implications of the
development of their new clinic and had to negotiate an additional line
of credit with Midwest.

After six months of operation, the group noticed that their collections
were falling. The hospital administrator, it turned out, was not trained to
handle professional fee billing and had done little to avoid the problem. No
insurance claims had been submitted during the six months. The physicians
were eventually forced to arrange a new short-term loan from Midwest
to cover their cash flow problem while they got their billing system back
on track. Midwest agreed to this new loan but with the stipulation that a
practice management consultant be engaged to guide the group in developing
its business systems. The physicians, however, feared the proposal was
a masked effort by Midwest to directly intervene in their affairs. They
countered the proposal by immediately hiring their own administrator. As a
result, the group did, during the next year, gradually stabilize its finances
and practice.

During the second year of operation, Midwest successfully recruited
the two new specialty physicians. However, it was quickly discovered that
the group could not honor compensation promises Midwest recruiters had
made. Yet another loan had to be arranged to permit this expansion of
the group. To this problem was added difficulty in recruiting additional
physicians to the group and enlisting area physicians into a network.

Midwest continued to financially bail the group out as needed. Inter-
estingly, if the group had any excess income, it was paid to the physicians
as bonuses rather than going toward accelerating repayment of the many
loans from Midwest. As a result Midwest gradually came to have a major
financial stake in the group's operation, which the physicians continued
to avoid acknowledging. Their independence was critical to them, and it
was rumored that they would prefer to declare bankruptcy than to concede
to a Midwest takeover or direct participation by Midwest in the group's
management or the management of their Deerfield hospital.

Analysis

This example highlights the danger the role of banker holds for hospitals and
medical groups. The physicians of Deerfield Family Practice wanted to have

their cake and eat it too. They wanted Midwest's considerable and ongoing financial support as well as their full autonomy. The case also points out the importance of sensitively but most definitely addressing the, at times, irrational need of physicians to feel independent.

11

THE ACQUISITION AND DEVELOPMENT
OF MEDICAL GROUPS BY HOSPITALS

Physicians are increasingly finding it acceptable to sell their practices to a hospital and then work for the hospital as employees. Hospitals are also finding it increasingly attractive to create new medical groups when doing so improves the hospital's competitive position. This chapter examines these trends and their advantages and disadvantages.

Changing Physician Attitudes
toward Working for Hospitals

Physicians are facing difficult times. Growing demands by the government, employers, and the public for cost-effective and higher-quality care are displacing the practice of medicine with administration. Practice costs combined with growing regulation are driving physicians to throw in the towel and look for alternative practice arrangements. The once great desire of physicians to have their own practice is fading. Having someone else worry about hiring staff, meeting the payroll, purchasing new equipment, billing and collection, and compliance with regulator policies and procedures and managed care contracting is beginning to look pretty good to many of them.

Earlier chapters discussed two reasons why physicians are moving in this direction. Physicians have difficulty accumulating capital to finance expansion and to cover liabilities. This problem, as noted, has led them to approach hospital administrators for financial help and to impose on them the role of banker. The second reason is the need for good quality managerial help that small groups often cannot afford. The growing disenchantment with independent practice is also fueled by changing personal preferences.

Changing Preferences of Younger Physicians

Physicians who are fresh out of residency are much less interested in coping with the many problems and risks associated with going into practice or buying a practice. There are a number of common problem areas that they wish to avoid.

To begin, they do not want to take the time to learn to manage their practice. This includes not wishing to spend the time to develop business plans; to deal with personnel problems, including resistance to change; to make hiring decisions; to deal with poorly designed operating procedures and information systems, including professional fee billing and collection; and to address facility management problems.

These time-consuming and often frustrating practice management obligations are further aggravated by the time new physicians must spend in building up a good reputation that develops their practice. First impressions are usually lasting ones. They must also spend time participating in medical staff functions both within and outside the hospital, including involvement in medical societies and hospital committees. And they must invest time in developing relationships with referring physicians and specialists who contribute to their practice such as radiologists, anesthesiologists, and pathologists.

To these considerations can be added all the anxieties, uncertainties, and frustrations of negotiating a buyout, which can involve hard-to-value accounts receivable and participation in real estate partnerships and other investments. A buyout or start-up is all the more difficult for physicians who carry considerable education debt and might not want to borrow large sums of additional money to buy or start a practice.

Yet another area of change lies in the changing lifestyles of younger physicians. They are not interested in being on call every night. They want to be able to take extended vacations, and they want to contribute to raising their children by having the time and energy to participate in school or athletic functions. They want to be able to go home at five and have dinner with their families rather than attending an evening medical group business meeting to figure out whether an HMO contract is advantageous.

Some new physicians are also not ready to settle down. The idea of locum tenens, where they are hired to fill in temporarily when a group or individual physician needs temporary help, is an attractive and exciting alternative to developing their own practice. And last, yet another phenomena that is beginning to change the profession is the increasing number of female physicians. They want to practice medicine and have a family. To do that, however, they must have a flexible practice situation. Group practice and salaried positions such as joining the staff of an HMO where patients are the responsibility of the organization offer male and female physicians the opportunity to have a lifestyle of their own choosing.

In sum, if physicians are going to have to work harder for lower reimbursement and receive less respect in the process, they want to see these losses replaced with a higher quality of life. Quality family time and more vacation and mobility to avoid feeling locked into one situation have become important considerations. These trends translate into opportunities for hospitals to offer employment arrangements that include guaranteed salary and benefits and a well-managed setting in which to perform their work. The effects of these trends are accentuated by a new trend developing among older physicians.

Retirement Considerations for Older Physicians

The changing practice trends for the young have created some difficulties for older physicians. These physicians traditionally planned to finance a portion of their retirement from the sale of their practice. The trend among young physicians toward becoming salaried employees of medical groups and other providers has undermined this traditional strategy. This growing realization has led them to look to hospital administrators for help. At the same time, hospital administrators have begun to appreciate that these physicians are important admitters and that the loss of their practice is a loss to the hospital. It is easy to see that the loss of a physician who admits 100 patients a year can have a noticeable impact on a hospital's bottom line when the marginal contribution per admission ranges from $2,000 to $3,000, depending on payer mix, case mix, and physician specialty and $3,000 to $5,000 for tertiary care hospitals.[1]

In sum, hospital administrators see a value in maintaining affiliated medical practices, while the physicians are beginning to feel that their hospital owes them something for their loyalty and are expecting the hospital to pay them back for their years of service by purchasing their practice.

Medical Group Acquisition

Chapter 10 discussed the partial involvement of hospitals in the ownership and direction of medical groups through joint ownership. The selling of a medical group involves the physicians in a process of relinquishing their control over their practice and becoming employees of the hospital and, therefore, subject to review and direction from the hospital's administration. This is a radical financial and psychological change for many physicians.

Selling forfeits autonomy and entrepreneurship and can be expected to be experienced as an anxiety-provoking loss. The agenda for the practice immediately shifts from the exclusive focus of supporting the physician's standard of living and needs for autonomy to serving the needs of the hospital, which includes ensuring a greater flow of patients to the hospital.

Hospital administrators must approach a buyout with caution so they do not give the impression that their motives are completely self-serving. The physicians involved should be patiently and sensitively helped to understand and accept that the sale means losing some if not all their authority over decision making, personnel matters, health plan participation, operations, and finances. They must also learn to appreciate that their expectations will become subordinated to the needs of the hospital, which might be struggling with external marketplace forces and operating issues such as reducing costs, increasing throughput, quality control, and utilization review.

A smooth transition in management is critical to successful future operation. The parties to the transaction should establish a board of directors composed of hospital administration and the selling physicians. It is important to note that in this board, as compared with a joint venture, hospital administrators have the final say in the decisions that are made. However, the board serves more as a communication medium that affords the physicians the important opportunity to give input and receive feedback on problems and issues while the hospital's leadership can use it to discuss direction and policy.

The sale and transition in leadership are the most difficult parts of this transaction for several reasons:

1. The purchasing hospital or organization must have an organizational structure that integrates operations and decision making and provides clear strategic direction.

2. The new owner must be prepared to operate the practice after the sale. The physicians and staff need a clear chain of command that is sensitive to their needs to avoid the immediate development of serious practice-threatening dysfunctions.

3. The hospital must be prepared to deal in an up-front manner with changes in compensation and benefits. It is critical to maintain the goodwill of the physicians and staff to be certain that the practice will continue to attract existing and new patients.

4. Care must be taken in implementing operating changes. Administrative changes can be depended on to create anxiety among clinic employees who might have a hard time understanding their ramifications.

These potential problem areas should be addressed during the buyout negotiations, which should also cover postpurchase management of the group, physician compensation, and the optimization of integration benefits.

Buyout Negotiations and Strategy

There are many scenarios that can lead to acquisition talks between physicians and their hospital. Regardless of the reasons for the sale negotiations, all issues must be fully examined and resolved before the acquisition is finalized. Some of the more critical points are discussed below.

The physicians involved are typically concerned about how the technical aspects of the acquisition will work, especially with regard to their personal stake in the practice. Administrators must appreciate that the physicians might have a significant portion of their retirement or personal net worth tied up in the practice's assets, so how they are valued and purchased is of great importance. Acquisition discussions should cover two points. First, they must address the process of acquisition, covering the legal, financial, and human dimensions of the transaction so that the physicians understand what will happen to their practice when it is acquired. Second, the parties need to have frank discussions about business and strategic planning so that everyone will share the same expectations about where the medical groups will be headed.

Among the more important legal and operating questions is how the hospital will organize its purchase. The hospital may choose to dissolve the practice's legal entity and move its staff and operations under its own structure. In this scenario the hospital can either handle the sale within its own structure or it can establish a separate entity to house the group's assets and manage and operate the practice. The route that the hospital takes depends on how many acquisitions are planned and how extensively it will become involved in medical group management.

An alternative purchasing plan is to take the group's assets into possession but maintain the practice entity, which then employs the physicians and staff. The assets purchased can include patient accounts receivable, buildings, equipment and furniture, and sometimes patient records. This approach is advantageous for hospitals that do not want to house medical groups within their own structure or do not have the vehicle to do so. This approach also saves the hospital from having to accommodate employment, benefits, and management needs within its existing structure.

Among the more important aspects of acquisition discussions is whether they are rushed. If the negotiations do not encourage thorough discussion and understanding and alienate physicians in the process, major operating problems can be expected to develop after the ink dries. The physicians might assume that the hospital will maintain the status quo in terms of how their practice is run. They may look at the new owner more as a banker that is only concerned with adequate collateral. They might also assume that if the practice is doing well that the hospital will leave it alone. The hospital administrator must make sure that the physicians understand that the hospital is going to protect its investment and will intervene in operations to resolve problems. However, even if the physicians involved acknowledge that they understand that the hospital will want to improve the practice and will intervene in decision making and operations, they might realize that they no longer have control only after the hospital acts to make change as the new owner.

Hospital administrators must also be sensitive to changes in the practice habits and patterns of the physicians themselves. Examples of changes commonly include stemming the loss of dollars in an HMO contract by cutting overutilization of services by primary care physicians, requiring physicians to work different or more hours, or asking them to perform additional tasks such as attending health fairs and participating in health screening programs on weekends. Other sensitive issues are decisions that affect the size and composition of the group, changes that physicians might feel interfere with existing patient care practices.

Hospital administrators should also make their financial objectives and limitations known to the physicians. They should make clear whether they intend to make a profit from the practice. The physicians must also understand how deep the hospital's pocket is in terms of spending to improve or expand their group's practice. This understanding becomes even more important if the hospital expects the physicians to contribute some of the financing through a reduction in their compensation.

Hospital administrators can facilitate physician understanding and appreciation by developing business and strategic plans that outline direction, including what needs to be improved and how. The hoped for result is a mutually agreeable game plan. If the process does not produce good results or identifies irreconcilable differences, both parties might want to reconsider the sale, restructure it, or perhaps consider a joint venture approach.

In sum, the important point is that the sellers are not just taking their money and moving on to something else. They will remain with the business that was once theirs. Hospital administrators must be open with the physicians during acquisition talks to avoid confusion and hurt feelings. By doing so, they will send a message to the physicians that they care about their needs, respect their values and expectations, and are committed to making the medical group a success.

Postpurchase Medical Group Management

Preacquisition discussions should include an evaluation of the current manager of the practice. As discussed in Chapter 10, the role of the medical group's manager can be important in completing negotiations. If the physicians have been pleased with their administrator's performance, they will be certain to protect the person despite negative evaluations by hospital administration. However, if the motivation for the sale is the result of internal political or financial problems, it is likely the physicians will not be too defensive if change is suggested. Discussions of change then focus on how it should occur.

One option is for the hospital-physician governing board to pursue the recruitment of a replacement. The board should develop a job description as well as answers to the questions posed below. This option allows the physicians the opportunity to participate in the process. However, the hospital might choose to limit their involvement in the selection process by only reviewing its choice with the physicians. The hospital might pursue this route out of fear that the physicians will want to hire someone who will side with them or who will not meet the qualifications of the position.

Another option is for the hospital to fill the position with someone from within the ranks of the hospital. This is a popular choice with hospital administrators as it permits picking someone who is a known quantity. It also provides upward mobility for employees and can save dollars by taking advantage of the skills of existing staff. However, hospital administrators must realize that bringing a medical group into a hospital's corporate structure does not mean it should be run like part of the hospital. Medical practice is very different and requires experience in a number of different areas unique to medical groups.

A last option is to use a management service. Considerable care must be exercised in making a selection if the buying hospital does not operate its own service.

Regardless of how the selection occurs, the hospital must see to it that a competent and diplomatic person is selected for this role. Candidates must know and understand medical group management, and they must be diplomatic enough to serve two masters, the physicians and the hospital administrator. The physicians, after selling their practice, will continue to insist on involvement in decision making. The group's new manager must be able to balance the interests of the physician and of the hospital to keep them working effectively together. Finally, the authority of the position must be established with the physicians and their staff. If the staff does not understand that the physicians have relinquished control through their deal with the hospital, they might be confused about who is in charge and unintentionally undermine the administrator. Physicians and hospital administration should take the time to meet with staff to explain what they have done and how it affects them.

In sum, hospital administrators must remember that even though the physicians are selling their practice, that does not mean that they no longer care about how it is run. One of the key events in developing a harmonious relationship is the decision who is to manage the group's business affairs.

Physician Compensation

Another major concern of physicians in selling their practice is whether they will lose income. The answer to this question lies in the motivation the hospital has in acquiring the practice. If the hospital is bailing out the practice by acquiring it (the banker role), then its management will probably be interested in being repaid. A rigorous approach to obtaining a return on its investment is to cap physician compensation, which can immediately confront them with the reality of their decision to sell their practice. However, hospital administrators might want to adjust payments to fit the available cash flow to avoid discouraging the physicians. If they cannot see themselves getting out from under the debt, they might lose the incentive to try and resent that the hospital is earning a profit from their services.

Hospital administrators should be frank with physicians about their compensation when outlining their financial objectives for the development or redevelopment of their group. If the plans require that the physicians take a cut in pay, then the hospital needs to explain this to every physician involved. Should the hospital decide to fix the salaries of the physicians, it must be careful about how it deals with workload assignment. The physicians will not readily accept a pay cut or a fixed salary while being asked to work longer shifts, to increase the number of patients seen per hour, or to drive ten miles to staff a new satellite office. A performance-based compensation methodology should be considered to provide optimum motivation.

Cost Saving Integration and Limitations

A number of important integration issues need to be discussed. The hospital's administration might wish to integrate the medical group's personnel and operations with those it already has to avoid duplicating management, personnel, and supply costs. An example is the use of the hospital's human resources department for recruitment, wage and salary administration, and benefits coordination. Hospital administrators should not hesitate to point out to physicians that they can offer many operating, time-saving, and cost-saving advantages. The following are some of these advantages:

- Assistance can be provided in locating physician backups to cover call, vacation, and continuing education schedules. These backups might, for example, come from another medical group that the hospital owns.
- Permanent physician recruitment services can be provided.
- Employee assistance programs and staff training and educational programs can be economically provided.
- Enhanced practice marketing and advertisement opportunities can be developed.
- Expanded data-processing capabilities, including on-line access to hospital data bases, can be provided.
- There are many areas of clinic operations where the hospital can supply assistance or savings through shared services or purchasing.

Yet another area of concern for physicians when integrating their practice with a hospital is the fear that their practice will begin to look like and act like a hospital. It deserves to be said again that medical practices do not operate like a hospital and therefore cannot be run like one. While there are areas where duplication can be eliminated and savings in purchases made, hospital administrators must appreciate that there are also limitations to integration. Even though both organizations have positions such as nurses, radiology and laboratory technicians, receptionists, secretaries, and billing personnel, they perform their roles differently. The data-processing needs of a practice are also different from those of a hospital. There also are many different forms, codes, and reporting needs.

In sum, the staff of a medical practice customarily experiences acquisition shock in changing from a stand-alone operation to membership in an organization many times its size. They might well feel lost about where they stand in the overall organization.

Establishing New Medical Practices

Hospital administrators can also develop their own medical groups. In this scenario, the hospital creates a new, fully owned and staffed medical group that employs physicians. There are important differences between developing a new medical group and acquiring an existing one.

This approach to networking is perhaps the easiest to implement since many of the buyout issues mentioned above are avoided. However, this strategy also possesses its fair share of risk and complexity. The following are some of the points to be considered in establishing a new medical group:

1. The hospital, by developing its own group, completely controls the decision making and implementation from the start.

2. The outlay of cash by the hospital might be less, and some undesirable assets might not have to be purchased.

3. The hospital can locate the practice exactly where it wants it. Convenience and good visibility are features important to the public.

4. The recruitment of physicians is easier because no buyin is necessary.

5. The hospital can create whatever type of practice it wants for the location as long as it does not step on the toes of other area physicians or appear to favor one group over another.

6. Hospital-owned and -operated medical groups appeal to young physicians who want to practice without the worries of buying into or managing a practice.

7. The hospital can plug the gaps in its medical staff by recruiting needed specialists and supporting them at these sites.

As can be seen from this list, the main advantage of developing a medical group is the speed and flexibility it offers the hospital. The development and implementation process becomes a "brick and mortar" project rather than a diplomatic mission. If the location does not compete with existing medical staff practices, the hospital should encounter little resistance and might actually be supported by area physicians if valuable new resources are provided that their patients currently do not have access to or have to travel considerable distance to access.

Conclusion

The ownership of medical practices by hospitals is a growth industry as hospital administrators strive to develop networks to expand their markets and revenues. However, this level of the integration of physicians is not without its complexity. Hospital administrators must approach target groups carefully, present a solid proposal that includes well-thought-out goals, and be prepared to persist as the physicians work through the meaning of the sale to them. It is critical that hospital administrators ensure that the physicians involved in the sale understand its consequences—the loss of the control of their practice to the hospital.

Case 11.1
Acquisition of the James Nelson, M.D.,
Practice by St. Mary's Hospital

Dr. Nelson (all names are fictitious), a 65-year-old family physician, had been the only doctor in rural Oak Grove for 35 years. However, Oak Grove was changing. Its population was increasing because of the opening of a new manufacturing plant. As a result, a new medical group had recently opened a clinic in Oak Grove, which was presenting Dr. Nelson with something new—competition.

Hospital services had been provided by a small 20-bed hospital that had a maternity unit and a surgical suite for minor surgical procedures. The hospital also operated an adjacent nursing home.

Tertiary care patient needs had traditionally been met at several other area hospitals. Metropolis, a large city 50 miles east of Oak Grove, had three major hospitals. Northside, a city of 50,000 located 25 miles to the north, had a large Catholic regional medical center (St. Mary's), which drew patients from a 50-mile radius. There was also another small hospital in Southland, 30 miles to the south.

Dr. Nelson managed his referrals to meet patient needs. Catholic patients were often referred to St. Mary's. Patients were referred to hospitals in Metropolis based on reputation, advertising, and a managed care arrangement with the new factory. Southland's hospital received few referrals from Dr. Nelson since residents of Oak Grove seldom traveled to Southland because of the poor road.

The growth of Oak Grove attracted the attention of area hospitals. A Metropolis hospital approached the new medical group for the purpose of acquiring it. The offer was eventually accepted. The purchase agreement included the group receiving coverage from other nearby hospital-owned practices, funding to develop specialty clinics, and a manager to run the group's practice.

At the same time, the hospital in Southland, not wishing to miss out on the new market, approached a large multispecialty group in Southland about opening a satellite clinic in Oak Grove. The group hesitated because it meant that they would have to build a clinic, which they were not financially prepared to do. However, the difficulty was overcome when the hospital stepped in to build the clinic space, which was then to be leased to the group.

These marketplace changes gradually became of increasing interest to St. Mary's management. They were becoming concerned that their referral pattern from Dr. Nelson was being slowly eroded by all the additional competition.

Several competitive strategies were considered. New physicians might be recruited to start a practice in Oak Grove. A medical group in Northside might be encouraged to develop a satellite in Oak Grove. The better idea seemed to be to acquire Dr. Nelson's practice. The medical director of St. Mary's knew that Dr. Nelson was planning on retiring and that he had not located anyone to purchase his practice. His practice accounted for 30 percent of all the admissions from outside Northside's immediate market area, and he was also a major referrer to specialists in Northside.

The director of outreach services at St. Mary's approached Dr. Nelson. Three main issues arose regarding the purchase: (1) the purchase of the clinic building, (2) the purchase of the practice, and (3) the development of an employment agreement to secure Dr. Nelson's services until a replacement physician could be recruited.

The first issue proved to be the most difficult to resolve. Dr. Nelson and his wife, who was also his business manager, were proud of their building and how well they had maintained it. They expected to receive a good price for it and its prime Main Street location. The management of St. Mary's was anxious about its purchase. The price was high, and if they were unsuccessful, they would be left owning a building that they did not need.

The second issue involved the purchase of Dr. Nelson's accounts receivable, office equipment and furniture, medical records, and goodwill. They needed to agree on a fair assessment of the value of his practice.

The third issue regarding his continued temporary employment did not prove to be difficult to resolve. He was to receive a salary, insurance, and benefits.

Negotiations spanned many months. The Nelson's consistently felt that the building and practice were worth more than what the hospital's administration thought they were worth. The Nelson's were not encouraged to change their minds since they also felt the hospital had a deep pocket and that St. Mary's owed them because of the their decades of loyal referrals.

A deadlock gradually developed. The administrator of St. Mary's suggested that he retain a management consultant at his expense to work with the Nelsons to help them develop an agreement. It was hoped that a neutral party would forestall the continued development of aggravation and mistrust on the part of the Nelsons. Dr. Nelson agreed to the hiring of a consultant.

The consultant hired a real estate appraiser from Metropolis to place a value on the clinic building. Next, the consultant worked to establish a fair value for the practice's assets. This proved to be difficult since Dr. Nelson's receivables were not maintained in a way that permitted ready access and analysis. Accountants were employed to prepare a schedule of receivables and an assessment of their worth. Meanwhile a representative of a medical supply company was engaged to assess the value of the furniture, equipment, and supplies. Dr. Nelson eventually agreed to the assessments. At this point the consultant returned to St. Mary's to discuss them.

St. Mary's administrator still thought the property appraisal was too high, and he hired his own appraiser. The second appraisal was not unexpectedly lower. Additional bargaining eventually yielded a mutually acceptable price. The hospital administrator accepted the accountant's and the supplier's assessments. At this point, Dr. Nelson raised one additional issue. He wanted his staff to have the option of continuing their employment. The hospital administrator agreed to this condition.

When the legal staff of the hospital began to draw up the contracts, a number of additional problems surfaced:

- The clinic building, it turned out, was built over the site of a gas station. Environmental regulations required that the ground be tested. If contamination was found, it would have had to have been removed at considerable expense before the sale could be finalized—a major cost that Dr. Nelson would have been expected to pay. Fortunately, the tests were negative.

- Maintenance employees from St. Mary's were asked to double-check the condition of the building. They reported it needed a new roof and heating system. While not eager to absorb these additional costs, St. Mary's administrator agreed to absorb them.

- Mrs. Nelson was asked to step down as administrator, which she agreed to do.

- St. Mary's attorney, to build in greater assurance that Dr. Nelson would fulfill his employment contract, asked that the payment for the purchase of the practice be tied to the completion of his obligation. Recruitment to a rural community was expected to be difficult and time consuming. Dr. Nelson agreed to half at closing and half at the completion of his employment contract.

- A final problem surfaced when St. Mary's hospital administrator met with his counterpart at the Oak Grove Hospital to discuss the sale. The sale of the practice did not turn out to be an issue; however, the status of Dr. Nelson's health and skills unexpectedly did become an issue. Patients had complained that they did not think Dr. Nelson could hear them. Dr. Nelson had a hearing aid that he did not wear. Other physicians and members of the nursing staff had also expressed concerns about his skill level. It was agreed that Dr. Nelson would be instructed to wear his hearing aid and that St. Mary's would pay to improve his skills.

The closing was successful.

Analysis

This case is an example of the complexity of dealing with changes in the marketplace and how much effort can go into the acquisition of a practice. It also highlights a number of the problems that hospital administrators can encounter in making a deal.

Note

1. T. M. Murphy and D. Hallock, "Group Practices Tie Hospital, Physicians Objectives," *Healthcare Financial Management*, August 1990, 21–28.

12

HOSPITAL-PHYSICIAN NETWORKING SUCCESS

This book has provided a comprehensive overview of the growing trend in hospital-physician networking. Some of the important points that have been made are as follows:

- The number of physicians in this country has grown tremendously. The popularity of practicing in medical groups has grown just as fast. The growth in the number and size of medical groups has made it important for hospital administrators to work with medical groups to address the needs of their community to remain competitive.

- The economics of providing health care has changed dramatically for hospitals and physicians. The FFS payment methodology has given way to DRGs, capitation, and now RBRVS. Reduced reimbursement has made it more difficult to cover increasing costs.

- The health care marketplace has also changed. Health care decision making regarding what to provide people and where, when, and how to provide it is being influenced by the payers, employers, and the government. At the same time, patients are demanding more convenience in seeking care and expect better outcomes for their health care dollars. Physicians and hospitals have found that they must compete to survive in the new health care delivery marketplace.

- Hospitals are responding to the new marketplace by diversifying. Decreases in the delivery of inpatient care have been compensated for by increases in outpatient care. Hospitals are taking advantage of new technology that permits many types of procedures that used to require inpatient stays to be delivered in the outpatient setting. Hospitals are also beginning to respond by building vertically integrated organizational structures that allow them to control more of the health care services being delivered.

- Hospital administrators are developing physician network strategies. They are encouraging their medical staff to become involved in the planning and development of their hospital.

- Hospital administrators are also beginning to appreciate the legal implications of networking. The government is concerned about price fixing and more recently with the possibility that physicians might be inappropriately referring patients to provider entities that they might in part own. Developing a legal and workable organizational structure that facilitates vertical integration between physicians has become a challenge.

- The task of choosing a partner for a joint venture or other networking arrangement is also a challenge for hospital administrators. It is important that they know the political structure and makeup of a target group as well as how its leadership functions. Medical group governance can vary from one senior partner running the group to the group being run by a committee that includes all the physicians. Each type of governance structure offers hospital administrators a different challenge.

- Hospital administrators must be prepared to assess the management and operating effectiveness of medical groups. It is critically important to understand what makes medical groups tick to understand the nature of the group's problems and what must be done to correct them. There is little reason to pour resources into a failing group that cannot be turned around.

- The offering of a medical group management service contract is a "foot in the door" opportunity for hospitals. Good quality management services are a first step in developing a networked relationship with a medical group. The important issue is for the hospital to ensure that good quality services are offered. Poor performance will undermine physician confidence and the ability to develop joint venture or ownership arrangements.

- Joint ventures and joint ownership of medical groups by hospitals creates a fully integrated marketing presence. Successfully dealing with issues of governance, financing, and management are the keys to success. Both parties must share common motivations and objectives to create a good partnership.

- The purchase of medical groups is yet another way that hospitals can ensure the loyalty of its admitting physicians. Voids in a hospital's market can also be filled by the development of new medical groups. Physicians looking for more flexibility in their lives and fewer headaches are finding these approaches to be acceptable new alternatives to starting out on their own.

In sum, the evolution of health care delivery and finance is providing hospitals and physicians considerable motivation to network if they are to survive and prosper.

Hospitals and Doctors Must Work Together

This book has discussed many of the reasons why hospitals and physicians should network. Some of the reasons mentioned are sharing expenses to take advantage of economies of scale, sharing strategic services such as planning, improving physician recruitment, and improving and expanding service opportunities. Most of the more important reasons for networking can be understood to fulfill three goals: (1) controlling the pricing of health care services, (2) improving the quality of service, and (3) maintaining the independence of health care providers.

Controlling the Pricing of Health Care Services

The pricing of health care services will remain negotiable between the consumers, the payers, and the providers as long as our health care system continues to operate on a free enterprise basis. However, as pointed out in this book, the nature of these negotiations is changing. Reimbursement methodology has changed from FFS to DRGs and RBRVS, and payers continue to look for new ways to structure payments involving multiple providers. Payers are beginning to want physicians and hospitals to join together to provide cost-effective care and to split a predetermined global payment for the care delivered. For example, global fee billing for surgical services might include all preoperative work, the physician's fee for the procedure, the hospital's charges for preoperative testing, operating room time, the inpatient portion of the care, and a reasonable number of follow-up office visits. Consolidated pricing promises to reduce administrative costs associated with the complexities of payers making payments to multiple providers. Consolidation also cuts the "middle man" out of the system for employers by permitting them to deal directly with suppliers of care rather than through an intermediary insurance company. And last, consolidation shifts the burden of allocating payments between the hospital and physicians to the providers. This approach is more than just a new idea. It is already beginning to be used by large employer health care purchasing groups.

If consolidated pricing is the wave of the future for reimbursement, then hospitals and physicians will be forced to work together to respond to contracts that call for global fees. Most importantly, they will have to agree on a method for pricing their collective service and splitting the resulting single payment.

The ability to put an entity together to collect and distribute consolidated payments is but one reason why hospitals and physicians must join forces in the 1990s. The 1980s saw the development of new incentives in the form of managed care. The 1990s might well become the decade of direct pricing intervention. Many politicians, corporate executives, and the public believe that the reason health care costs continue to skyrocket is that the prices providers charge are unreasonable. Thus far this sentiment has led to payers applying major discounts to their reimbursements and to an accelerated trend in the use of antitrust legislation to limit physician-hospital cooperation. As a result, physicians and hospitals have been blocked from benefiting from the advantages of collective bargaining during contract and reimbursement negotiations, with the outcome that they have lacked the clout to countervail the power of payers to unilaterally impose reduced payment structures. This must change if hospitals and physicians are to maintain control of their services. The good news is that some change is already foreseeable in the antitrust position. The legal climate, as mentioned in Chapter 6, is beginning to change due to the actions of large employers who want to deal directly with providers to create consolidated care. This new trend is encouraging the government to reconsider its position and allow the development of multiprovider organizations if they can demonstrate an ability to reduce costs and maintain quality.

In sum, the control of the pricing of health care services is a dynamic arena that contains many powerful players on all sides of the bargaining table. The only certainties are uncertainty, change, and the eventual response of providers to the suppression of their autonomy, interests, and reimbursement.

Improving the Quality of Health Care Delivery

Hospitals and physicians who argue for fair payment must demonstrate to payers that they are receiving good value for their money. Regulating the quality of health care has emerged as the latest challenge to managers of medical practices and hospitals. To date, the sacred nature of the practice of medicine has not required physicians to demonstrate that the care that they provide is of high quality and cost effective. Peer review is the closest thing to monitoring the efficacy of the health care that they deliver. However, during the 1990s that is going to change.

Employers, who are paying larger percentages of their operating budgets for health care, are beginning to require providers to produce evidence that they are getting their money's worth. Physicians and other health care providers are beginning to be treated like any other vendor. Manufacturers who subject their parts suppliers to quality specifications are beginning to apply the same principles to physician and hospital services.

Networked physician-hospital organizations offer both parties the structure to accomplish this task. Quality and efficacy assurance, to be effective, must include the full spectrum of the care delivered, which ranges from office visits to surgery, physical therapy, and home health care. A joint effort must be mounted to accomplish the required monitoring. Hospitals and physicians must combine their data bases to provide a complete health care delivery picture for health plan enrollees.

This trend will eventually lead to the issue of who will conduct the reviews—hospitals and their medical staffs or the staffs of health plans and employers, who will use their own outcome measures. This issue becomes even more important to physicians if the review is concurrent and offers the threat of interfering with the delivery of daily care.

It is therefore obvious that it is critical for providers to demonstrate a willingness and ability to assume this new responsibility or risk the threat of losing additional control of their services. There are also two additional reasons why hospitals and physicians must combine forces to monitor quality. First, providers cannot easily satisfy requests for quality assurance information from the health plans, insurance companies, employer groups, and the government. The purchasers are not likely to be able to agree on a standard quality assurance format and data base. As a result, the imposition of many different standards and information formats will create yet another expensive and time-consuming regulatory bureaucratic layer that the industry can ill afford to absorb. Voluntary development of a self-regulatory process will forestall this outcome.

Second, any review of physician decision making must protect the physician-patient relationship. Invasive payer policies and procedures that require in-depth knowledge of the condition of and treatment plans for patients can risk alienating the patients as they lose confidence that their desires for privacy are being respected. Once again, a self-imposed system creates a win-win outcome for physicians and their patients.

In sum, medicine should try to remain an industry that polices itself. Outside, businesslike review of care would create new costs, depersonalize physician-patient relationships, and invade the patient's right to privacy. The development of hospital-physician networks might be the only way of responding to these new demands.

Maintaining the Independence of Health Care Providers

The final reason for hospitals and physicians to network is their desire for independence. Our health care system will very likely undergo major changes as the debate over access and cost continues. Some of the proposed changes, if implemented, will dramatically affect how health care is delivered and how it is controlled.

Providers are already on the defensive when it comes to reducing the rate of rising costs. The RBRVS represents only the latest effort of payers to redistribute reimbursement among medical specialties and to cut payments. Cost containment has led hospitals and physicians to accept lower reimbursement while quality control issues have led payers to demand more say in how providers do their work. In sum, hospitals and physicians are locked in a struggle with payers for control of the health care industry.

This struggle for control is forcing hospitals and members of their medical staffs to circle their wagons in the hope of maintaining control. The age of independent physician medical practice (in particular solo and small group practice formats) might be reaching an end. Physicians and hospitals are losing their independence, not to each other but to employers and health plans who see owning these providers as the ultimate way to control their costs through controlling the practice of medicine.

Their control will mean that physicians will lose some of their privilege of independent judgment in their practice of medicine. At an extreme, some fear that physicians will be reduced to the level of highly trained technicians who have their work supervised by their employer's quality control experts. Hospital administrators also risk losing their prerogatives in designing their service menu to compete with other hospitals. Competition is seen by payers as creating costly duplication of services. Payer certificates of need could conceivably emerge for hospital facility and service expansion.

In sum, hospitals and physicians must put themselves in a position to have some say in how the health care system evolves. Working together will permit them better control of their destiny by offering purchasers reasonable prices, good access, and service as well as the data needed to assess the quality of care.

Conclusion

This book has provided the reader a sweeping but thorough overview of the constantly evolving health care delivery industry. From the vantage point of the early 1990s it appears that the industry will evolve toward ever greater networking of hospitals and physicians to protect their remaining control of health care decision making and reimbursement while at the same time providing more cost effective and better quality care, which is necessary to avoid nationalization of the industry.

Hospital administrators have been forewarned throughout the book to be prepared to know and understand physicians and medical group management. This is critical if networking success is to be achieved without excessive investments of money and time. The authors hope that they have contributed to this better understanding and helped to point the way toward being effective networkers in the growing integration of the health care industry in the 1990s.

INDEX

Accounting system, assessment of, 115
Acquisitions (of medical groups by
    hospitals), 159–65, 172; buyout
    negotiations and strategy, 161–62;
    case study, 167–70; cost savings of,
    164–65; difficulties with, 160–61;
    legal arrangement of, 161; medical
    group manager and, 163; physicians
    and, 158–64; transition operation,
    160, 163–64, 165. *See also* Medical
    groups, management; Safe harbors
Administration of marketing. *See*
    Marketing
Advertising, 61
Alternative structuring (of hospital-
    physician relationships). *See*
    Hospital-physician relationships
American Medical Association (AMA),
    64; definition of medical group,
    5; predictions for medical groups,
    14–15
Ancillary services, assessment of,
    110–11
Antitrust, 79–80
Appointment system, assessment of,
    105–15

Business systems (of medical groups):
    accounting and fiscal administration,
    115; ancillary services, 110–11;
    appointments and scheduling, 103–5;
    internal marketing issues, 6–8;
    managed care contracting, 117;
    management service agreements for,
    123–24; medical group manager,
    118; medical records, 111–13;
    personnel administration, 108–10;
    productivity, 116–17; professional
    fee billing, 114–15; purchasing and
    inventory management, 113–14;
    reception and registration, 105

Capital formation, physicians and, 24
Capitation payment methodology,
    19–20; hospital-physician structuring
    for, 25
Case studies: Metropolitan Sports
    Medicine Center, 151–53; Midwest
    Hospital Corporation and Family
    Physicians of Deerfield, P.A., 153–
    56; Midwest Hospital Corporation
    and Northland OB/GYN, P.A.,
    130–33; James Nelson, M.D., Prac-
    tice and St. Mary's Hospital, 167–70
Centers of excellence, 46–47
Centralized scheduling, 104
Climate control system, assessment of,
    107
Collaboration (of hospitals and
    physicians), 15–16, 56, 74, 129–30,

ABOUT THE AUTHORS

Todd S. Wirth is the administrator of a large orthopedic surgery group and a health care consultant in Minneapolis, Minnesota. He has served as the chief operating officer of University of Minnesota Clinical Associates, as department administrator of the Department of Family Medicine and Community Health at the University of Minnesota, and as assistant administrator of the department of medicine at the University of Missouri–Columbia. He has also served as the chief administrative officer of U Care Minnesota, a Minnesota health maintenance organization. Mr. Wirth has published numerous articles on medical practice management and managed care. He is a nominee of the American College of Healthcare Executives and an active member of the Medical Group Management Association. Mr. Wirth received his undergraduate and master's degrees in public administration from the University of Missouri.

Seth Allcorn is Associate Dean for Fiscal Affairs at the Stritch School of Medicine, Loyola University at Chicago. He has also served as the administrator of the department of medicine at the School of Medicine and Dentistry, University of Rochester, and of the University of Missouri–Columbia School of Medicine. Dr. Allcorn has published a number of books and chapters and more than 50 papers regarding hospital administration, medical group management, and the psychodynamics of organizations. His latest books are *Workplace Superstars in Resistant Organizations* and *Codependency in the Workplace*. He is a member of the Medical Group Management Association and the International Society for the Psychoanalytic Study of Organizations. Dr. Allcorn has received two degrees in business administration and a Ph.D. in higher and adult education.